"Even people who eat a healthy, ill. That's why this book is need us to live wisely while we are s but also by caring for ourselves a and, if necessary, I want to die w⌐ ... you do also, then start reading."—From the foreword by **Michael Greger, MD**

"I really didn't think that a book about the mortality of vegans would be so beautiful and empowering, but it is. It's full of sound advice, wisdom, and resources that give you clarity and courage in spite of a culture that prefers to avoid the truth of mortality. It reminded me that it isn't until we accept our own inevitable death that we can fully live and love ourselves and others as the interdependent, imperfectly perfect animals that we are. This is the most important book I've read in a long time, and it will add so much to the vegan cause, community, and canon."—**Marisa Miller Wolfson**, Writer/ Director, *Vegucated*

"**Even Vegans Die** knocked my socks off with its integrity. I was thrilled to read a book by three powerful women telling it like it is! It is so refreshing and easy to read. It is filled with sobering truth and firm, kindhearted advice reminding us that even our fellow vegans deserve compassion."—**lauren Ornelas**, Founder/Executive Director, Food Empowerment Project

"Overflowing with compassion and practical wisdom, this book tackles sobering issues of illness, caregiving, death, mourning, and isolation that all people, vegan and not yet vegan, will inevitably confront. Everyone should read this book and reflect on Carol, Patti, and Ginny's caring advice for living, and eventually dying, well."
—**Lori Gruen**, author, *Entangled Empathy*

"A real-life guide to, well: real life, which includes death—despite one's diet, attitude, or how many times one hears, 'You don't look your age.' Addressing a real problem in the vegan world—that being sick or, heaven forbid, shuffling off this mortal coil somehow makes us 'bad vegans'—this thoughtful and knowledgeable trio of writers help us in their honest and forthright book to deal wisely with the fact that our days are numbered, and to live with vibrancy and purpose every day we've got."—**Victoria Moran**, author, *Main Street Vegan* and *The Love-Powered Diet*

"Brilliant and inspiring! Carol, Patti, and Ginny have filled a gap in vegan literature with a guide that is as practical as it is powerful. **Even Vegans Die** helps us navigate many of the challenges we and our loved ones confront as we age. I learned so much from this wise, wonderful, and immensely important book."—**Mark Hawthorne**, author, *A Vegan Ethic: Embracing A Life Of Compassion Toward All*

"**Even Vegans Die** is a must-read for vegans—an essential and honest reflection on topics that most of us choose to ignore. This book tells us why it is so important for the vegan community to face and embrace these issues."—**Anya Todd, MS, RD**, vegan dietitian and animal rescuer

"At sanctuaries, we know better than anybody that everybody dies. We also know that people are most likely to hurt themselves or others when they mistake themselves for superheroes. **Even Vegans Die** offers a refreshing and essential antidote to all-too-human delusions of invincibility, while also arguing (accurately) that the vegan and animal advocacy movements will become more effective by embracing diversity, including diversity of body size and health experience. As a bonus, the book offers practical advice alongside astute analyses."—**pattrice jones**, author and co-founder of VINE Sanctuary

"As a chubby, vegan culinary instructor and cookbook author, I'm hyper aware of the fact that I don't fit the bill for selling veganism ('But you're not skinny'). And I cringe when some of my culinary students misunderstand that a vegan cooking class is different from a weight-loss cooking class. In an attempt to make veganism sexy, there's a pervasive message that vegans are skinny, disease-proof, and should look 30 when they're 70. That's not fair to the incredibly diverse vegans I know—of all sizes, shapes, races, ages, gender identities, and religions—and it sure doesn't help the animals. This book is important and it's done just right. It's a tool for vegan activists to speak pragmatically about the health benefits (and myths) of a plant-based diet. It's a guide for dealing with the realty of health, illness, and, ultimately, death: death of the people we love, as well as our own. And it's a call for rational compassion. Hats off to the dynamic trio of authors who tackle this difficult topic with kindness, truth, and hope.—**JL Fields**, author *The Vegan Air Fryer* and *Vegan Pressure Cooking*

"The benefits of a plant-based diet and a healthy lifestyle are underutilized and underappreciated, yet concurrently to some they represent a moral high ground as an impenetrable shield defying risk, chance, and even death. To be sick or overweight or in any way unrepresentative of an ideal body is deemed unclean and immoral and the fault always lies on the individual. But the research that outlines the benefits of a vegan diet also shows us that disease and death are a part of our lives beyond diet and lifestyle. A range of body types has always existed and will continue to exist and to expect otherwise is detrimental to our collective health. **Even Vegans Die** is here to remind us that snake oil is not vegan and in order to do the most good we have to accept this reality and act accordingly."
—**Matt Ruscigno, MPH, RD**, co-author, *No Meat Athlete* and *Appetite for Reduction*

"Why is a title as obviously true as **Even Vegans Die** so provocative? This much-needed book from some of the vegan movement's most compelling thinkers not only provides insights into this question, it also offers a wide range of practical advice on how to better care for ourselves and our community—and why it's critically important to do so. Eschewing perfectionism, denial, and blame, the authors present a care-centered lifestyle and model of effective activism based on discerning realism and profound inclusivity. The result is an empowering set of theories and recommendations that embolden people of conscience to create more deliberate lives and more enduring legacies."—**Dawn Moncrief**, Founding Director, A Well-Fed World

"**Even Vegans Die** tackles hard questions related to illness, death, mourning, and caretaking, especially as they impact those who care about animals. The result is a book that brings a new dimension to these issues, exploring them in ways that help us become better advocates for animals, for our fellow vegans, and for our own legacy."—**Marc Bekoff**, author, *The Animals' Agenda: Freedom, Compassion, and Coexistence in the Age of Humans*

⚜ Even Vegans Die ⚜

*A Practical Guide to Caregiving,
Acceptance, and Protecting
Your Legacy of Compassion*

———

Carol J. Adams, MDiv, Patti Breitman,
and Virginia Messina, MPH, RD

———

Lantern Books ● New York
A Division of Booklight Inc.

2017
Lantern Books
128 Second Place
Brooklyn, NY 11231
www.lanternbooks.com

Copyright © 2017 Carol J. Adams, Patti Breitman, and Virginia Messina

This book is not intended as a substitute for the medical advice of a licensed physician. The reader should consult with their doctor in any matters relating to personal health. To find a health professional who can provide individual nutrition counseling for vegans, visit http://www.eatright.org/find-an-expert.

Printed in the United States of America

Library of Congress Cataloging-in-Publication Data

Names: Adams, Carol J., author. | Breitman, Patti, 1954- author. | Messina,Virginia, author.
Title: Even vegans die : a practical guide to caregiving, acceptance, and protecting your legacy of compassion / Carol J. Adams, Patti Breitman, and Virginia Messina, MPH, RD.
Description: New York : Lantern Books, 2017 | Includes index.
Identifiers: LCCN 2016055043 (print) | LCCN 2017001696 (ebook) | ISBN 9781590565537 (paperback) | ISBN 1590565533 (paperback) | ISBN 9781590565544 (ebook) | ISBN 1590565541 (ebook)
Subjects: LCSH: Terminal care. | Vegans--Death—Social aspects. | Veganism.
Classification: LCC R726.8 .A33 2017 (print) | LCC R726.8 (ebook) | DDC 616.02/9—dc23

LC record available at https://lccn.loc.gov/2016055043

Don't try to live forever, you will not succeed.
—playwright and vegetarian George Bernard Shaw

In loving memory of
Rynn Berry, Jay Dinshah, Bill Harris, Marti Kheel,
Dave Middlesworth, Tom Regan, Lisa Shapiro,
Sam Simon, Mark Sutton, Shirley Wilkes-Johnson,
and other beloved vegan activists

⊰ **Contents** ⊱

Part 3: A Vegan's Guide to Death and Dying

⊰ **Foreword** ⊱

Michael Greger, MD

Wait! What? The author of *How Not to Die* is writing a foreword to a book titled *Even Vegans Die*? Yes, and here's why.

Let me remind readers that my book is entitled *How **Not** to Die*, not *How to **Not** Die*. It's an important distinction because until the biology of aging is sufficiently teased out, we're all going to die. Vegan or not.

Just as seat belts reduce risk of serious harm or sudden death, so a healthy diet can reduce risk of many conditions and diseases—ranging from the merely inconvenient to those causing premature death and extreme disability. People who buckle up are less likely to suffer harm than those who don't. People who eat well are more likely to live longer than those who don't. We wear seat belts not because of some guarantee that we're not going to die in a fiery car crash, but because we're rational and want to decrease our risk. But even people who wear seat belts can be seriously harmed in a car crash. Even people who eat a healthy, plant-based diet can get seriously ill.

That's why this book is needed. Carol, Patti, and Ginny emphatically believe in the power of a healthy vegan diet for reducing risk of premature death. They also suggest that in recognizing that we can't reduce that risk to zero, we improve our lives. We become better advocates for a healthy lifestyle and a more humane world, and we make better decisions about how we will die. Carol, Patti, and Ginny teach us to live wisely while we are still here, not only by eating well, but also by caring for ourselves and one another.

Even Vegans Die offers valuable insights and practical answers to questions that I am frequently asked to address. In fact, I see our two books—*How Not to Die* and *Even Vegans Die*—as a great set of bookends on your shelf. To start with, you need to know how to eat and live as healthfully as possible to enhance your chances of staying well. But we all need to know how to deal with illness in ourselves and others, and how to make the best decisions about treatment, caregiving, and end-of-life issues.

Even Vegans Die should be helpful for folks of all stripes. The personal stories from vegans who are dealing with chronic illnesses are especially instructive and they highlight the importance of addressing body shaming, disease shaming, and even the stigma of choosing medical care within the vegan community. This book's compassionate perspective on illness and dying will resonate with everyone, vegan or not.

And I wholeheartedly agree with the recommendations regarding our bodies and science: Sign up to be an organ donor and even to donate your body to science when you die. What better way to continue your life of compassion after you're gone?

So yes, I am happy to write the foreword of *Even Vegans Die*. I want to live well and, if necessary, I want to die well, too. If you do also, then start reading.

⊰ Introduction ⊱

Facing Your Own Mortality Can Enhance
Your Life and Advocacy

FACING MORTALITY IS HARD, AND VEGANS ARE NOT ALONE IN choosing avoidance and denial in thinking about our own deaths. But we believe that our time on Earth will be more meaningful and more rewarding when we fully and consciously acknowledge that it is limited.

We are going to make the case that it is urgent as *vegans*, to our activism and our lives, to acknowledge that we die. We're going to talk about how facing our own mortality builds a stronger and more compassionate community of animal advocates, puts us in greater control of our own health, and even ensures that our efforts for animals will not end when we die. It allows us to ensure a legacy that includes caring for animals, and it lets us shape the way we want to be remembered.

People come to veganism for many different reasons. But regardless of those reasons, many end up with a misguided faith in the ability of a vegan diet to keep them healthy. Too often, vegans view illness, and especially a terminal illness, as a personal failure. We feel shame about falling ill ourselves, and may participate in blame when other vegans become sick. But we are better activists, and a much more supportive community of activists, when we recognize that vegans, including those who do everything "right," can still get sick.

It's true that a vegan diet can reduce our risk for a number of chronic diseases. But no healthy diet or lifestyle offers an ironclad guarantee against disease. Some vegans get cancer and diabetes. Some vegans have heart attacks. When we fail to recognize this, we risk alienating people from our vegan community. We miss the opportunity to provide care and support to other vegans. We also deny some vegans the right to advocate for animals. Instead of building up our community, we diminish it.

Believing that veganism is a panacea for all human ailments sets up veganism to fail. Recognizing that vegans can get sick—sometimes seriously so—and that none of us is immortal makes us more compassionate. An honest perspective on the limits of veganism when it comes to health lets us support rather than judge, broadens our community of activists, and encourages us to be more effective on behalf of animals.

There are also personal benefits that accrue when we come face to face with our mortality. Doing so, allows us to prepare for the difficult questions that face vegans who are seriously ill. As a vegan, you've most likely spoken out against animal testing. Or perhaps you've even suggested to others that Western medicine is overhyped and that a plant-based diet is the best defense against disease. These and other views can be suddenly challenged when you are faced with an illness that is most effectively treated with chemotherapy or other allopathic drugs. What would you do if you had a serious illness that could be treated only with a drug that had been tested on animals? We're going to encourage you to think about these and other challenging questions.

And then there are the practical considerations. If you rescue animals or have turned your home into a safe haven for "difficult" animals, who will care for them if you die suddenly? When we talked to vegans about this, many of them said, "I'm still young," i.e., "Nothing is going to happen to me yet." Vegans who are 30, 40, 50, 60, and 70 said this to us. Here's a tragic fact: the most frequent calls to many animal rescue groups come from family members after someone has died. "Come NOW and get the cat, the dog, or we will have them euthanized."

What if you get sick and are unable to make decisions about your own care? Do you want heroic interventions if you are dying? Do you want to be buried after you die? Do you eventually want your animals to be buried with you? Do you want your remains treated in a way that protects wildlife habitat?

These are vital, even urgent questions that we are going to explore in this book. We're going to share practical advice about creating a vegan community that is more inclusive and that cares well for vegans who are sick. We address facing your own illnesses with compassion and creating a legacy that will long outlive your body. We'll look at how acceptance of our death can be braided into our activism and our lives.

In our book *Never Too Late to Go Vegan* we talked about how embracing a vegan ethic is a way to feel empowered at a time of life when people often perceive themselves to be losing power. Now, we want to take the next step. Overcoming denial of your mortality, facing it, and acknowledging it is another way of feeling empowered, of gaining control over something that can feel frightening.

Even vegans die. Let's see how we can use our knowledge of this basic fact of life to make us better champions for animals and one another now and in the future.

A NOTE OF WELCOME TO READERS WHO ARE NOT VEGAN
When we first started brainstorming for this book, we had several goals in mind. We wanted to explore myths about diet and disease that can lead to shame and blame in the vegan community. We aimed to look at how these issues affect choices about health care among vegans as well as plans for when we no longer are around. And we wanted to provide a model for compassionate caregiving and advice on making things easier for those we will leave behind.

But as the manuscript evolved, we recognized that non-vegans (or veg-curious folks) might also pick up this book. If that's you, we welcome you. We think that you may find that much of what we talk about is helpful to you even as a non-vegan. Our guidelines for caregiving, thoughts on mourning, and advice for creating a will apply universally. We've presented a perspective on diet and disease that is likely to resonate with anyone who feels embarrassment or shame when they get sick with a chronic illness. Likewise, the problem of weight stigma extends far beyond the vegan community. It's an issue of importance for everyone.

Finally, we expect that as you read this book, you'll encounter some views that deepen your understanding of what veganism is all about. In fact, we think you'll find that much of what underscores a vegan ethic resonates with what you already believe and how you want to live your life. ✎

Part 1

Vegan Health

The Myths and Realities

Even Vegans Get Sick

WE SEE IT EVERY DAY ON OUR FACEBOOK, TWITTER, AND Instagram feeds, in blogs and books.

Pictures of older supermodels who credit a vegan diet for their flawless, ageless looks. Before-and-after photos of people who say the pounds just melted away when they went vegan. Testimonials from those who've never had a cold since they stopped eating animal foods. No doubt you've heard that a plant-based diet will immediately clear up your skin, and that once you begin eating only plants, you'll have boundless energy you've never experienced before.

It's no wonder vegans can start to feel invincible when we fill our shopping carts with whole plant foods. On a recent trip to Costco, glancing at their basket piled with quinoa, peanut butter, extra virgin olive oil, pinto beans, chickpeas, hummus, lemons, and frozen blueberries, Ginny's husband remarked, "If diet really matters, we should live to be 150."

Diet does matter, of course. (And Ginny's husband, who has a PhD in nutrition, knows that very well.) But the extent to which your diet can protect your health isn't always clear. More significantly, nutrition experts don't always agree on exactly how we need to eat to be at our healthiest.

Are you surprised? Within the vegan community, there's a fair amount of faith in the miraculous benefits of a diet that includes only whole plant foods. Not just that this is the only healthy way to eat, but that it's guaranteed to keep you healthy.

Many people do experience major health benefits when they adopt a diet built around minimally processed plant foods. Replacing animal foods with whole plant foods and healthy fats is almost assured to reduce your saturated-fat intake, for example, which in turn protects against heart disease. If you've struggled with elevated cholesterol, a vegan diet is an excellent approach to lowering it. Replacing meat with beans in menus boosts potassium intake, which helps lower blood pressure. And yes, research has even found that eating a healthy plant-based diet can give your skin and your immune system some extra protection. This might slow the aging process and it might give you considerable defense against viruses.

There's a lot to celebrate and share about the health benefits of vegan diets. It's the promises and guarantees we need to be careful about.

How We Talk about Diet and Health

Chances are you know at least one person who has long defied the odds. You know the type—he smokes, eats meat three times a day, hates vegetables, and doesn't exercise. And he's never been sick a day in his life.

Or how about the opposite situation, the person who does "everything right"? This is the vegan whose plate is always loaded with fruits and veggies. She meditates and exercises. And she still ends up with cancer.

It doesn't make sense in view of what we know about the kinds of foods and dietary patterns that prevent and cause disease.

But when we start talking about diet and disease, we have to tread carefully around words such as "cause" and "prevent."

You can improve your odds of staying healthy and avoiding life-threatening chronic illnesses. How you eat, along with other lifestyle factors, can certainly affect your risk of becoming ill. But there is nothing you can do—at least based on what we know right now—to ensure that you never get sick.

Medical research has provided us with much information about how to eat for a long and healthy life, and for the most part it points us toward a plant-based diet. But there are also gaps and inconsistencies in the research that leave us with questions. Also, when we look around the world, it's pretty clear that the populations that live the longest, healthiest lives eat a *plant-centered* diet. That is, they eat a diet that is packed with plant foods and low in animal foods. None of these populations is vegan.

Information about the health of vegans was lacking for a long time. But we're starting to get some insight thanks to two large ongoing studies. The EPIC–Oxford Study in England includes around 2,600 vegans. The Adventist Health Study-2 in North America includes nearly 8,000 vegans among its subjects.

Both of these studies assessed dietary intakes among vegans and also among meat eaters, lacto-ovo vegetarians, and semi-vegetarians (those who eat meat less than once per week) enrolled in the studies. The researchers are following all of the groups to track rates of different diseases. So far, findings suggest that vegans, on average, are slimmer than meat eaters and even than semi-vegetarians and lacto-ovo vegetarians. Not surprisingly, vegans also are at lower risk for type 2 diabetes and for hypertension. Vegans appear to be less likely to develop certain cancers.

But there have been a few surprises, too. Although, in the U.S., vegan men have a lower risk for heart disease, vegan women don't appear to enjoy the same protection. Research from the United Kingdom showed that vegans had a reduced risk for dying from heart disease, but risk was even lower for lacto-ovo vegetarians and pescatarians.

We don't know exactly what that means. The research in this area is still new and our knowledge is imperfect. We don't know the exact dietary recipe for eliminating chronic diseases. In fact, we don't even know if such a recipe exists. All kinds of other factors affect risk of illness, including how well we are able to deal with stress and depression, our social life, physical activity, and the immediate environment. Certainly, genetics plays a role.

We can do "everything right," based on what we know now, and still get sick. Even where vegans have a clear advantage, the benefits don't extend to every single vegan. Some vegans have hypertension. Some have diabetes. Some have elevated cholesterol. In interviewing people as part of the research for this book, we talked with vegans who suffer from cancer, heart disease, hypertension, multiple sclerosis, diabetes, asthma, lupus, Crohn's disease, irritable bowel syndrome (IBS), arthritis, thyroid disease, depression, and osteoporosis. We heard as well from vegans who have struggled to lose weight.

Vegans also get colds and the flu. Vegan skin can break out. And some people never notice any change in their energy levels when they go vegan. Although it can be disappointing to know that a vegan diet may not cure every problem you have, it's also reassuring to know that your vegan diet hasn't failed you every time you get the sniffles, or even if you become sick with something much more serious than a cold.

Knowing a vegan with a chronic disease such as cancer, heart disease, or diabetes can give you a sense that the world has spun off its axis. It challenges what we believe about diet and disease. The only explanation is that the person must have done something wrong. They didn't do veganism right—that's why they got sick. Or they were "cheating" on their vegan diet.

We might explain to ourselves that they ate processed foods. Or they went vegan too late in life to reap its true benefits. Those kinds of beliefs help us avoid an uncomfortable truth: We don't have complete control over our health. This is especially true when it comes to complex diseases like cancer.

Diet and Cancer

Cancer starts with a mutation in a single cell. By the time it progresses to full-blown disease, a lot of things have to happen, though, and the body has plenty of opportunities to undo the damage or prevent it from progressing.

Diet may play a big role throughout the process. For example, antioxidants in plant foods can prevent mutations from happening in the first place. Or if cancer cells are already growing, compounds in plants can inhibit processes that allow tumors to spread. Some can even prevent formation of the blood vessels that feed tumors.

Based on what we know about diet and cancer, it's reasonable to expect that people eating plant-based diets should have a lower risk for this disease. Some evidence suggests that they do.

In the Adventist Health Study and the EPIC–Oxford Study, vegans had lower rates of cancer than people who include animal foods in their diets. But their risk wasn't zero; it was about 15–20 percent lower compared to meat eaters. Being vegan doesn't mean you can't get cancer.

So is it that we need to be eating a particular type of vegan diet? Is it that we aren't eating enough broccoli or we're eating too many veggie burgers? Maybe. But we don't actually know. One of the best and most authoritative resources on diet and cancer is a report from the World Cancer Research Fund and the American Institute for Cancer Research. Their expert panels have reviewed all of the research on diet and cancer and ranked foods, nutrients, and dietary patterns according to the strength of the evidence.

For example, for breast cancer the panels determined that there is *persuasive* evidence that alcohol raises risk and also evidence that obesity *probably* does the same. After that, the evidence gets a whole lot weaker. It's limited (or inconclusive) regarding a host of dietary factors, including fats, fiber, dairy foods, and specific dietary patterns. Likewise for colon cancer: There is persuasive evidence that red meat raises risk, but little compelling evidence that other factors are protective.

It might mean that diet is simply not powerful enough to prevent all cancers. Or it may be that we need more research in order to determine which dietary factors are most decisive. But before you throw in the towel on diet and cancer, it's worth noting that the report mentioned above recommends eating a plant-based diet as one significant guideline for reducing cancer risk. A plant-based diet is widely recognized as a good way to reduce cancer risk. It just can't promise to eliminate risk entirely.

WHY WE USE THE WORDS *OVERWEIGHT* AND *OBESE*
When we talk about body size and body shaming, words fail us. They really do. As much as we recognize that how we discuss body size often reflects bias and promotes stigma, language hasn't caught up. The medical community uses the words *overweight* and *obese* as diagnoses, based on BMI (body mass index). But because BMI doesn't consider body composition or any health parameters, we sometimes end up attaching more meaning to it than is warranted. It doesn't actually tell us how much fat is on a person's body and it doesn't tell us anything about the individual's health.

It's simply impossible to take the judgment out of the terms *obese* and *overweight*. Even when used without any intention of judging, there's a pejorative aspect to the words. They convey the idea that there's something wrong with your body, that you are different from the norm, from what is healthy and ideal. This opens the door to shame, blame, stigma, and discrimination.

In her book *Fat Shame*, Amy Farrell writes: "Women in the United States today face a far different standard regarding body size than those of other times or other cultures." She also notes glaring uses of fat stigma among vegan organizations and publications. We find it, too, from blogs to health professionals, from activist campaigns to books.

Farrell points out that stigmatizing of "fatness" and juxtaposing it with the "fit" or the "vegan" or the "civilized" body ends up justifying discrimination and inequality. It also keeps us from thinking clearly "about health issues within this national and international anxiety regarding the 'obesity epidemic.'"

What words, then, should we use in this book? The problem is that we don't really have better words. Some activists who are tackling the issue of body shaming have embraced the word *fat* to describe themselves. For others, this remains a painful and loaded term. Research suggests that people have different preferences about terminology and this makes the issue even more complicated. It leaves us with no good way to talk about body size. We've opted to use the words *overweight* and *obese* in this book since these are the scientific terms used in the medical and nutrition communities.

In discussing the issue of body shaming, which urgently needs to be addressed in the vegan community, we recognize that our language remains imperfect.

Even Vegans Get Heart Disease

It's much easier to study the relationship of diet to heart disease than to cancer. We can do intervention studies by feeding people a particular type of diet and looking at what happens to their cholesterol and triglyceride levels and even the health of their arteries. As a result, we have a better idea of how people need to eat in order to prevent heart disease. Eating lots of whole plant foods and unsaturated fats and avoiding saturated fats from animal foods appears to be the best approach. We have good reason to believe that a healthy vegan diet is a powerful plan for lowering risk for heart disease. But will the right diet *eliminate* your chance of getting heart disease? If so, do we know what that diet looks like?

Some books, articles, and blog posts suggest that we can end heart disease with the right lifestyle approach. The evidence suggests otherwise. We can dramatically lower risk for heart disease, but we are not at the point where we know how to completely prevent or cure it. Although some popular vegan health advocates have suggested that vegan diets that are very low in fat can reverse heart disease, no well-controlled studies show this. We have only anecdotal and observational information from the individual practices of some doctors. In the world of evidence-based nutrition, this doesn't count for much.

One exception is the Ornish study that was published in 1990, which showed remarkable reversal of heart disease with a plant-based diet combined with exercise, smoking cessation, and stress management. The diet wasn't quite vegan—it included very small amounts of nonfat dairy and egg whites. And because the study incorporated so many health-supporting factors (stress management, for example, is especially impactful when it comes to heart disease), it's hard to determine just how much of an effect diet alone had.

But at the very least, the study shows that a comprehensive heart-healthy plan that includes a near-vegan diet had a remarkable effect on heart disease. More than 80 percent of the subjects who followed this Ornish plan saw a reversal of their atherosclerotic plaques. That's incredible. But it's also necessary to note that not everyone improved. Is it because they cheated? Is it because the diet isn't completely vegan? Is it because the diet is too low in fat—given that we now know that higher-fat plant foods offer protection against heart disease?

It could be any of those things. It could also be that some people—for whatever reason—are at such high risk for heart disease that a healthy diet will only go so far in giving them protection. Or it could simply mean that we still don't know exactly what type of diet and lifestyle, if any, gives total protection against heart disease.

In a 2014 blog post, vegan activist and English professor Laura Wright said, "I have grown to believe that none of us, no matter how well trained, knows much about what makes us work and what makes us break, particularly when things break in the wrong people at the wrong time." This was five months after Laura, a long-time vegan and distance runner, suffered and nearly died from a massive heart attack at age 43. She was, she wrote, "The kind of person who should be a poster child for all the things that one should do to avoid having a heart attack."

Her heart attack turned out to be the result of a genetic predisposition that led to a spontaneous coronary artery dissection (SCAD), a condition that affects otherwise healthy women. It causes a spontaneous tear in the lining of an artery. Even a vegan diet is not likely to protect against a condition like Laura's. In fact, it's not even clear how much a vegan diet protects against heart disease in women generally. We don't have much information about vegan diets and heart disease, but evidence suggests that vegetarian diets (including both lacto-ovo and vegan patterns) are less protective against heart disease in women than in men. Since postmenopausal women are more likely to develop heart disease than men, we know that there are factors affecting risk that may have nothing to do with diet. And even though men seem to reap heart-protective benefits from plant-based diets, the research on these benefits is not consistent or conclusive. Vegan men can get heart disease, too.

Vegans and Diabetes

There's a strong genetic component to diabetes, and although being overweight raises risk among susceptible people, it can actually occur in people who are at normal weight, too. Risk factors for diabetes include not just poor diet, obesity, and a sedentary lifestyle, but also factors that can be more challenging to manage, like stress and depression.

The importance of diet can't be overstated, though, and choosing a vegan diet is a smart way to lower risk for diabetes or manage it if you already have this disease. Among subjects in the Adventist Health Study, vegans were 60 percent less likely to develop diabetes than meat eaters over a two-year period. Research from doctors with the Physicians Committee for Responsible Medicine has also found that a vegan diet is beneficial in managing diabetes. Whether you can actually reverse diabetes through a healthy diet is more complicated. In writing this book, we spoke with a number of vegans who were controlling their diabetes on a vegan diet but who hadn't reversed it. Others were diagnosed with diabetes *after* they went vegan. One told us that she deals with criticism from all directions. Her non-vegan family says that eating all of those carbs gave her diabetes, whereas some vegans have said that she's not "vegan enough," or she would never have gotten diabetes.

Again, this is a disease about which we don't have a complete understanding regarding prevention or treatment. People from certain ethnic backgrounds—African American, Latinx, Native American, and South Asian—are at much greater risk for this disease. It's not true that diet alone is always sufficient for control of diabetes.

The bottom line: A vegan diet is likely to lower risk for diabetes and can be useful in managing it. It's not a guarantee against diabetes.

Vegan Diets and Depression

Like cancer and heart disease, depression is a chronic illness. Evidence is mounting to show that diet can play a role in some types of depression. In particular, inflammation is thought to make depression worse. Since research suggests that vegan diets are associated with lower blood levels or markers of inflammation, going vegan could have a positive impact on your mood. In fact, a few studies have linked vegan or vegetarian diets with improved mood. Simply eating more fruits and vegetables could be beneficial, too.

But we do need to tread carefully here. Considerable stigma is attached to depression, and it's a disease that sometimes is complicated by shame and blame. It's fair to say that eating a healthy diet may improve some symptoms of depression, but it's simplistic to think that going vegan will automatically cure it. Depression is more complex than that, or at least some types of depression are.

In fact, whereas we vegans may have the advantage of our diet, some of us could still be at risk for depression. Some evidence exists that vegans are generally more empathetic (which isn't especially surprising), and there's also evidence that empathy raises risk for depression.

Depression is a serious disease that not only affects quality of life, but can raise risk for other conditions, like heart disease. It can be useful to take advantage of as many tools as possible to fight depression, which include exercise, therapy where appropriate, and a healthy diet. But even with all of those approaches at our disposal, some vegans who are depressed may benefit from medication, which has been shown to be most effective for those with severe and also with chronic low-grade depression. There's no shame in suffering from depression and no shame from doing whatever you have found to be most beneficial in dealing with it.

Even Vegans Get Wrinkles

When supermodel Christie Brinkley turned 61 a few years ago, one blog post from a national animal rights group highlighted her flawless appearance by saying: "Wowza! Stunning Christie Brinkley, 61, credits vegan diet for her youthful looks." There's no doubt about it—Christie Brinkley in her sixties looks lovely, just about as lovely as she looked in her thirties in fact. But the idea that her vegan diet is completely or even mostly responsible for this is, to put it bluntly, nonsense.

Christie looks the way she does because she was born with a particular set of genes and because she has the time and money to nurture and protect her looks. She has not had cosmetic surgery, but by her own admission has done lots of other "modern-technology stuff." A quick look at any online celebrity magazine reveals that many (or most) aging celebrities look great. This is true whether or not they are vegan (most of them aren't), because they have the same advantages that Christie has. Airbrushing, photoshopping, and other techniques can also alter their image in print.

Dietary choices can affect how you age. Antioxidant-rich plant foods, for example, may help to ward off some of the effects of sun damage. The phytoestrogens in soy foods may help prevent wrinkles to some extent. But promising vegans that we'll all age as beautifully as a supermodel is flat-out dishonest.

Not only is it one more way in which we set up veganism to fail, but it also perpetuates cultural ideas that are ageist and sexist.

There's nothing wrong with wanting to take care of your skin. Nor is there anything wrong with enjoying makeup or hair coloring. In fact, vegans who use these products are helping create a demand for products that aren't tested on animals. But we should be realistic about how far we can go with diet and makeup when it comes to warding off aging. And we should always be cognizant of the fact that wrinkles, saggy necks, and gray hair—just like chronic illnesses and body size—have nothing to do with our relationship to veganism.

Efforts to retain a youthful look reflect an understandable desire to hold onto the power that diminishes as people, especially women, age. We suggest there are other ways to be powerful, and veganism itself is one of them. It empowers us in ways that can't diminish as we age.

Vegan Diets and Dementia

Risk for chronic diseases such as heart disease and cancer increase with age. But of all the conditions associated with aging, none is quite so fearful as dementia. It's normal to get a little more forgetful as you get older, but that's different from dementia, which is a chronic progressive disease that interferes with daily functioning.

The most common dementia is Alzheimer's disease (AD). It involves degeneration of brain tissue and formation of plaques, called amyloid beta, in the brain. The cause of Alzheimer's isn't clear, but it appears to be the result of some combination of genetics, lifestyle, and environmental factors.

The apolipoprotein E (APOE) gene is involved in late-onset Alzheimer's. Having one particular form of this gene, called APOE ε4, raises risk for AD. It doesn't mean that a person who has this form of the gene will definitely develop AD. Nor are those who don't have the gene a hundred percent protected.

Another common type of dementia is multi-infarct dementia. This is caused by small strokes in the brain and can be related to high blood cholesterol and high blood pressure.

Although we don't have much in the way of good research on rates of dementia among vegans, it certainly seems like those rates should be lower. Research tells us that vegans often have less inflammation in their bodies, lower cholesterol, and less insulin resistance, all of which can protect against development of dementia. Diets high in saturated fat and trans fats have been linked to greater risk for AD. Plant foods are rich sources of antioxidants that may help make the blood–brain barrier less permeable to proteins that contribute to beta-amyloid accumulation. Provided you are including sources of vitamin B_{12} and long-chain omega-3 fats in your diet, there is every reason to believe that eating a healthy vegan diet lowers risk for dementia along with other chronic diseases.

This is one more example wherein it's not clear that healthy eating can completely overcome genetics. Or at least we don't know what we need to do in order to protect completely against dementia. And therefore vegans are not immune.

It's one more reason why some of the other issues we discuss in this book—such as drawing up a will and contemplating arrangements for pets—are just as necessary for vegans to understand as for those who eat less healthfully. We know that our healthy lifestyle gives us an edge against all kinds of chronic illnesses, including dementia. But we know, too, that there are no guarantees in life for vegans or anyone else. Any of us could lose the ability to make appropriate decisions.

Food May Not Always Be Medicine:
The Case of Multiple Sclerosis

There's no doubt that diet can be a powerful way to reduce risk for chronic diseases, particularly diabetes and heart disease. But some conditions continue to be a little bit of a mystery. Multiple Sclerosis (MS) is one of them. We know of several vegans with this disease, and it's a diagnosis that's understandably hard to fathom when you are living a healthy lifestyle.

MS is an autoimmune neurological disease associated with inflammation. As MS progresses, the myelin sheath surrounding nerves is destroyed and nerve fibers are damaged. It's a disease that affects young people, usually diagnosed between the ages of 20 and 50, and is far more likely to affect women than men. Right now, MS is incurable, but certain drugs can slow its progress.

Research from several decades ago suggested that diets low in saturated fat and high in omega-3 fats could slow the progress of MS. Widely known as the Swank Diet, after the neurologist who developed it, this approach greatly limits saturated fat and therefore limits animal foods. Contrary to popular opinion among vegans, though, it was not a vegan diet. The meal plan also allowed regular consumption of chicken, fish, and nonfat dairy products. Daily consumption of cod liver oil was recommended.

Although Dr. Swank claimed good results from his diet, it was an observational study and did not have a control group. To date, no evidence supports the use of the Swank Diet for MS. There's also no evidence that a vegan diet lowers risk for MS or controls symptoms and progression of the disease.

One thing that may reduce risk for MS is adequate vitamin D through supplements or exposure to the sun. But this isn't a vegan or vegetarian issue since these sources of vitamin D are available to everyone. Beyond this, there's currently little evidence for a link between diet and MS.

This may change as more research is conducted. But it's also possible that some conditions are simply not affected by a vegan diet.

The Importance of Self-Care

Stress is a normal part of life; everyone experiences it from time to time. For animal advocates, though, the stress associated with caring and compassion can become chronic and overwhelming. It can lead to compassion fatigue and burnout, making you less effective in your advocacy. It also takes a considerable toll on your health.

Although taking time out for self-care may feel selfish, it isn't at all. Protecting your own health and well-being puts you in a much better position to care for others and advocate for animals. Eating well and exercising are especially important, but they may not be enough to ward off stress and illness. Here are a few additional things that may be helpful.

Get adequate sleep. Sleep deprivation can increase inflammation in the body, making you more susceptible to illnesses, including depression.

Try to expose yourself to outdoor light. If possible, get outdoors for a short walk or other activity every day. In Japan, the therapeutic effect of being outdoors is called *shinrin-yoku*, which translates to "forest bathing." Don't worry if you don't live near a forest; simply being outdoors is good enough.

Engage in one or two daily practices that help relieve stress. These might include meditation, prayer, writing in a journal, or simply talking to a friend. Creative pursuits like playing a musical instrument, knitting, or painting can be helpful, too.

Find your community. Being involved with others who share your concerns and goals can be therapeutic and uplifting. If you don't know other vegans where you live, find them online.

Avoid online spaces that make you stressed and unhappy. These may be accounts that show graphic images of animal suffering or engage in body shaming or in shaming people whose habits they disagree with.

Being Proactive about Health Goes beyond Prevention

One of the damaging results of a vegan sense of invincibility can be complacency. In 2013, we published *Never Too Late to Go Vegan*, inspired in part by a conversation that Carol observed on Facebook. A group of post-menopausal women were discussing their shock at discovering they had osteoporosis. They thought they were protected by their vegan diet.

When vegan activist Sarah Kramer was diagnosed with breast cancer, she told her followers:

> I plan on blogging about this. Why? Because I want you to get serious about your breast health. I go for regular mammograms and I do self–breast exams after my period every month. If it wasn't for the regular monthly self-exams I wouldn't know how lumpy my thick breasts normally felt and that this particular lump felt different than the rest.

Catching disease early—whether it's blood pressure that is starting to creep up, early signs of insulin resistance that can be a warning sign for diabetes, or an unusual lump that appears out of nowhere—makes it easier to treat the problem. In addition, regular screening for early signs of cancer are just as imperative for vegans as anyone else. According to the National Cancer Institute and the American Cancer Society, three types of screening can reduce risk for death from cancer and are recommended. These are tests that screen for colon, breast, and cervical cancer. (Recommendations for PSA testing are currently under review, but this test has been shown to detect prostate cancer in its early stages. Talk with your health care professional about whether you should have this test.)

We urge you to consider incorporating these screenings into your life, if you have not already done so.

GUIDELINES FOR CANCER SCREENING

SCREENING FOR COLON CANCER

Beginning at age 50, any of the following four tests can be used to detect both cancer and precancerous polyps (which means they can prevent cancer):

- Flexible sigmoidoscopy every 5 years, or
- Colonoscopy every 10 years, or
- Double-contrast barium enema every 5 years, or
- CT colonography (virtual colonoscopy) every 5 years

The following tests can detect cancer but not polyps:

- Yearly guaiac-based fecal occult blood test (gFOBT), or
- Yearly fecal immunochemical test (FIT), or
- Stool DNA test (sDNA) every 3 years

SCREENING FOR CERVICAL CANCER

As for screening for colon cancer, Pap tests can prevent cancer. They can detect abnormal cells that can be treated before they turn into cancer.

Women ages 21 through 29 should be screened with a Pap test every 3 years.

Women ages 30 through 65 should be screened every 5 years with Pap and HPV co-testing or every 3 years with a Pap test alone.

SCREENING FOR BREAST CANCER

Although there is a longstanding controversy about whether women need to have mammograms between the ages of 40 and 49, there's widespread agreement that women over the age of 49 should have regular mammograms, either annually or every other year.

The downside to earlier screening is that younger women have denser breasts, which makes mammograms harder to read. It means you're more likely to have a false-positive result—something that looks suspicious but turns out not to be cancer. There's also a greater risk of over-treatment, since small, slow-growing cancers that might never have caused any problems can be detected.

The upside is that earlier screening increases the odds of detecting and treating cancer. The age at which you should begin having mammograms is something to discuss with your health care provider.

SELF-EXAMS

For women, being aware of changes and lumps in your breasts is critical. It doesn't mean you need to do a formal self-exam, since simply being familiar with the way your breasts feel has been found to be just as effective.

For everyone, it's a good idea to keep track of changes in moles on the skin. Depending on individual risk, regular skin exams by a dermatologist may be recommended.

If you believe that a vegan diet places a shield of protection around you, it's easier to miss early signs of a potential illness. In a way, accepting that you can get sick could help to protect you from getting seriously unwell.

Setting up Veganism to Fail

By eating a healthy vegan diet, avoiding tobacco, getting regular exercise, and managing stress, you can presume that you are doing your best to protect your health. But it's wise to accept that it may not be enough. Doing so eliminates the burdens of blame and shame that the hyping of veganism may encourage if you or others become ill.

So why so much hype and promise about vegan diets? Mostly we do it for the best of reasons: because we want to save animals. Most people want to look and feel great and many want to lose weight. If we can make them believe that a vegan diet delivers all of those benefits and more, it seems like animals will benefit.

But there's a downside to this. We set up veganism to fail when we make promises about a vegan diet that we can't keep. If someone gets sick, or doesn't lose weight, or their diabetes doesn't go away, then the very thing we promised about veganism has turned out to be untrue.

Dietitian Anya Todd, who is a vegan and an animal rights activist, gives talks at vegfests and other events. She's forthcoming about the fact that she herself lives with a chronic disease, fibromyalgia. Although she has seen that vegans sometimes want to hear only good news about veganism, she believes that it's valuable for all of us to manage expectations about health: "It's important for people to realize that a vegan diet is not a disease cure-all. Believing that it is can be problematic in encouraging people not just to go vegan, but to stay vegan if they are thinking only about their health and not seeing the results they expect."

Losing faith in the benefits of veganism is one reason that people return to eating animal foods. So this promise of long life and perfect health can backfire and end up failing the animals.

It also betrays our fellow animal advocates. It creates a closed community: vegans who get sick may no longer feel they have a place. And the consequences of this can have serious repercussions for our work for animals.

There's another reason why we're tempted to view veganism as a panacea against disease. It gives us a sense of control over our health and also over the uncomfortable fact that we will eventually die—because it's scary to realize that our control is limited or, in the case of death, nonexistent.

None of this is to say that you should give up on a healthy, vegan lifestyle. How you eat, exercise, and manage stress are all valuable to maintaining wellness. Healthy habits can improve how you feel now and lower your risk of chronic disease in the future. They might very well give you a few extra years of life. And it's pretty great that a vegan diet can be part of this health-promoting package when it's also the way we eat to protect animals and the environment.

But accepting that vegans can get sick is a key part of our successful activism. It promotes more realistic expectations about veganism that may actually help people stay vegan. Knowing that a vegan diet isn't a panacea for all ills frees us up to make realistic and informed decisions about treatment if we do get sick.

It also allows us to be more compassionate to vegans who are ill. Just as importantly, it allows us to face our own illnesses with compassion.

⊰ 2 ⊱

How Shame and Blame Affect Our Health and Our Advocacy

 F OR THOSE WHO BELIEVE THAT VEGANISM PROVIDES UNIVERSAL protection against getting sick, then an "ill vegan" is a contradiction in terms. It's not supposed to happen, yet here you are, proof that it does. If this can happen to you and you're vegan, might this also happen to other vegans? One of Carol's 60-something friends remarked, "Every time I hear a vegan is sick, I panic." Why does she panic? Because she accepted the theory that veganism was a panacea and now she has to confront that it isn't so. Are we actually mortal? Yes we are. And when we fail to acknowledge that, we open the door to shaming people about their illnesses.

Disease Shaming

Vegans who experience shame for their illness are likely to feel alienated from the vegan community. Shame may make them afraid to share their diagnosis with others. At a time when a person is in most need of emotional support, they may be afraid to ask for it for fear of being judged.

Some may be reluctant to admit that they've chosen conventional treatment for their cancer instead of trying to

24

cure it using more "natural" means, like a whole foods vegan diet. Susan Voisin, who writes the *Fat Free Vegan* blog, explains her reluctance to initially share her cancer diagnosis with readers:

> My image of myself as a healthy person who never took pills and was confident her vegan diet would protect her from anything—that image took a pretty big hit. I've been worried about "coming out" as a vegan with cancer for fear that non-vegans would see it as proof that a vegan diet "doesn't work," and that some vegans would skewer me for resorting to traditional medicine.

Her fears speak directly to what we mentioned in chapter 1 about the danger of holding veganism up to too-high standards, those of a magic elixir against disease. The danger intensifies if we view a vegan diet not just as preventive, but as treatment for diseases. Although a vegan diet can be a wonderful approach to treating heart disease or type 2 diabetes, it's never been shown to cure cancer. Nor has any other dietary approach.

Stories about people who cured their disease with diet may seem inspiring, but they can be harmful if they convince others to delay potentially beneficial medical treatment. Eric Polsinelli spent thousands of dollars and many years seeking a treatment for his Crohn's disease, almost costing him his life. It was an ileostomy that finally helped him heal. Another vegan, Jo Anna, wanted to avoid medications in treating her psoriatic arthritis. She said that changing her diet helped a lot with some of the symptoms, but that, "the real help was, sadly, when I started HUMIRA injections. Big guns medicine."

According to Apple CEO Steve Jobs' biographer, Jobs "deeply regretted" his decision to try alternative therapies for nine crucial months after he was diagnosed with a pancreatic tumor. We have no way of knowing if this cost Jobs his life. We do know that these alternative therapies didn't save it.

When Helpful Advice Turns into Shaming

When someone is ill there are all kinds of things you can do for them: helping with pet or child care, preparing some meals, cleaning up their kitchen, or running errands. If they want company, just sitting quietly with them can also be a form of care (see chapter 4).

Suggesting your favorite cure for cancer or other life-threatening diseases may or may not be helpful. It's an area in which you need to tread carefully. When Sarah Kramer was diagnosed with breast cancer in 2013, she received scores of tips on approaches for treating it. She was grateful for them. She researched the options and went with conventional treatment, while also incorporating alternative practices into her routine.

Not everyone wants that advice, though. Particularly for those whose diagnosis is grave, what seems helpful at first blush can simply turn into another form of disease shaming. It places another burden on sick people, this idea that if they do the right thing—juicing, raw foods, an alkaline diet, or a low-protein diet—they can cure themselves.

On top of being sick, they now need to worry about whether they are making their illness worse through their food choices. This can be a source of both anxiety and guilt two burdens that people with cancer don't need to take on. And chances are—if they have any interest in changing their diet to improve their prognosis—they'll find the information they need on their own.

We know of one woman who expressed anger toward her sister who had stage IV ovarian cancer. She wanted her to engage in "proactive, positive thinking" as a way to fight the cancer rather than simply to submit to it. But sometimes, the person with cancer is ready to submit. Advice about unproven cures may shift attention and energy away from things that might serve the dying person better—like spending time with loved ones, getting their affairs in order, making peace with their mortality, and employing whatever energy they have on enjoyable pursuits.

Blaming Yourself

One vegan who was diagnosed with cancer before the age of 30 said that it wasn't surprising to her. She had been overweight and ate a junky diet, so it was no wonder she had gotten cancer. But cancer in your twenties is unusual even among people who eat the worst diets.

When you are struck with a frightening disease, it's easy to start doubting yourself and your choices. It's human nature to look for an explanation—part of our desire to take control. Here is Susan Voisin again on her cancer diagnosis:

> Why did I, a vegan who tries to eat healthy, get cancer when no one else in my Standard American Diet–eating family has ever had cancer? What had I done wrong? Had I eaten too few nuts? Too little cilantro? Not enough flax seeds? BPA? Soy?! I worried that I had caused my cancer by never being able to get to my goal weight and stay there, that I didn't exercise consistently, that I had had only one child late in life and that I hadn't breastfed her long enough. I was blaming myself, and I had a lot of help from the Internet.

Vegans who struggle with understanding why they got cancer sometimes must come to terms with the fact that there is no explanation—or at least not one that we can know. Lisa, who was diagnosed with breast cancer, said that her greatest struggle has been within herself:

> I eat healthy, I'm very active, etc., etc . . . and I got cancer.
> I am determined to do everything I can to help myself get
> and stay cancer free, but I thought I was already doing so
> much. Can I be "more" vegan? Why wasn't that "enough"?
> It comes up in conversation with others—"but you were
> always the healthy one." Yeah, well healthy people still get
> cancer.

Although self-blame can be damaging, it doesn't mean that you can't let a health scare turn into a wake-up call about dietary and other lifestyle habits. A healthy diet packed with fruits and vegetables and other whole plant foods has been linked to improved prognoses for people with cancer. Gabe Canales was inspired to launch the nonprofit Blue Cure to promote prevention through a healthy lifestyle after he was diagnosed with prostate cancer at 35. His efforts are laudable and it's hoped can make a difference in the lives of men who are at risk for the disease. At the same time, it's a wise strategy to avoid letting language about prevention turn into self-blame. On the *Huffington Post*, Gabe wrote, "I was just another heedless American when, at 35, I was diagnosed with prostate cancer, supposedly an 'old man's disease.' But poor lifestyle and diet choices had encouraged and enabled my cancer."

Again, it's not clear how much these factors contribute to cancer at such a young age. It's also imperative to avoid the stress and anxiety that can accompany an attempt to start doing everything right for your health. If you are dealing with a chronic disease, especially one that has a demonstrated relationship to diet like heart disease, it's wise to take a look at your lifestyle and start working toward improvements. But it doesn't mean that you need to monitor every single bite of food because of how it might affect your cancer. Eating a vegan cupcake now and then is not going to make or break your long-term survival.

When Body Shaming Morphs into Disease Shaming

Our society already shames people who are overweight even when they are perfectly healthy. Add a chronic disease into the picture and the shaming escalates. For many people with obesity, it can quickly dissolve into self-blame.

We need to approach the subject of body weight and disease risk with both compassion and an honest evidence-based point of view. Yes, compelling evidence tells us that being obese can raise risk for cancer, diabetes, and heart disease. But it doesn't mean that everyone who is overweight is unhealthy. Nor does it mean that people with obesity who develop these diseases caused their own illness. They might have gotten sick either way. Furthermore, not everyone who goes vegan or "does all the right things" regarding diet and exercise can achieve a slim body. It's true that epidemiological studies suggest that vegans are less likely to be overweight or obese. But despite what you may read on the Internet and in books and magazines, there are no long-term studies showing that any particular vegan diet guarantees permanent weight loss for everyone. Some vegans do not lose weight when they go vegan and some gain weight—even when they are eating the very low-fat type of vegan diet most often touted for weight loss.

It's not clear why long-term weight management is more difficult for some than others. It could be an inherited "thrifty gene" that favors fat deposits or differences in brain circuitry regarding feelings of "reward" from eating.

Shaming people about their weight promotes weight bias and is damaging to the psychological well-being of our fellow vegans who are overweight. It encourages chronic dieting, something that can be harmful to health in the long run. Dieting changes metabolism in ways that boost hunger and affect calorie use that may make it even more difficult to manage weight.

Constant struggles with weight promote stress and depression. Both are risk factors for chronic disease. Sometimes, accepting your current weight as your "best weight" can be one of the healthiest things you can do. The Canadian Obesity Network defines your "best weight" as *whatever weight you achieve while living the healthiest lifestyle you can truly enjoy."*

Choosing to live a healthy lifestyle that includes good food choices, exercise, and stress management, and taking body size out of the picture, could very well do more to protect against illness than another attempt to slim down.

Putting Aside Shame and Blame Builds a Stronger Activist Community

At the core of a vegan ethic is our effort to widen the circle of compassion to include animals. Shaming and blaming people for their body size, appearance, or for having a disease belies that compassion. There are many people in our vegan community who are suffering and who need support from fellow vegans. Janet is a vegan with lupus. She says:

> Having a chronic disease is hard enough. It's isolating. People are afraid you will die and don't want to get close. People get tired of you cancelling. People stop treating you like you're a person. Add to that the stigma of being vegan and not being the picture of health, even if you've done all the right things, is just unbearable.

A constricted and restrictive view of who is allowed to speak for animals reduces the impact of our vegan community. The shame and blame that often accompany obesity or chronic disease has the unfortunate result of turning animal activists into non-activists. When Ginny asked her blog readers how living with a chronic disease or with obesity affected their relationship to veganism, she heard one particular response over and over: I don't engage in activism because other vegans have made me feel ashamed of my weight. Lisa, a San Francisco native who has been a vegan and animal advocate for nearly thirty years, says, "I do what I can but I want to do more, much more, and would if not for being self-conscious about being fat." She said that her long history of physical problems that produced weight gain had led to fellow vegans actually challenging her vegan status.

Scott, a 34-year-old vegan writer and editor, recently posted to Ginny's blog to say that it's difficult to connect with animal advocates who "rely on the narratives of health and weight loss to get people interested in the vegan message. Some of those advocates are openly hostile to meat eaters who are overweight. That hostility may not be specifically directed my way, but it is still deeply felt by overweight vegans like myself."

Caela, who was diagnosed with type 2 diabetes several years after going vegan, says that she doesn't interact much with local vegans. "I feel like an outcast due to my weight and medical conditions. I feel that there is such a push to show that veganism is so healthy and that all vegans are slim that there's no room for me."

Finally, making vegans feel ashamed about illness denies them the opportunity to celebrate and acknowledge the importance of their impact. Rachael has Crohn's disease:

> I have heard of people with Crohn's who have gone vegan and it's solved their problems. At times I feel sad that the same has not been true for me. However, I am at least lowering my risk of other health conditions and I feel better emotionally to think that even when I am doing nothing because I am too ill, that I am still helping by choosing to eat vegan.

Often, those who identify strongly with their own veganism find that others identify them by their disease. They suffer both stigma and an inability to claim their own identity. It is heartbreaking to think that activists are being pushed aside from a movement that they care deeply about. It's also a great loss to the animals, who need as many voices as possible. In fact, they also need the unique voices of vegans whose efforts have been either inspired or buoyed by their own experience with illness.

Rather than retreating from the vegan world, some have found new inspiration in chronic disease. Eric Polsinelli was already a vegan when he was diagnosed with Crohn's disease and eventually had to have a permanent ileostomy. Because no resources were available for vegans with ostomies, he started his own website, which provides, among many other resources, information about how to find vegan ostomy supplies. His contribution is unique and is strengthened because of his own experience.

Ellen is a long-time vegan who sometimes worries that people will draw incorrect conclusions about the relationship of a vegan diet to skin health because she suffers from adult acne. But over the years, she's found that more often than not her food choices help to start conversations and bring awareness about veganism. She says, "Perhaps my imperfections have become a kind of filter? It's my experience that there are many compassionate people who are willing to look past the surface to see the real issues at hand. Maybe these are the people most ready to consider a change?"

Research from the field of psychology tells us that people are more open to messages when they come from people they perceive as being similar to them. This alone speaks to the need for a community of activists that celebrates diversity. That diversity must go beyond gender, sexual orientation, and skin color to include people of different sizes and people whose experience with health differs. Breaking down the boundaries of our vegan community is the only way we will be able to build a vegan world.

Part 2

Caregiving as Vegans

❧ 3 ❧

A Vegan Ethic of Care

A S WE WERE WRITING THIS BOOK, A TRACTOR-TRAILER CARRYING 160 pigs to a slaughterhouse overturned, killing 40 piglets outright and leaving many others injured. Some tried to run away; others screamed from the pain. An injured animal cannot be killed to become food for humans, so activists and an animal sanctuary cofounder requested that the injured piglets be released to them to receive medical care and continue to live. But the slaughterhouse employees killed the piglets instead. Of course, this would have been the decision of the slaughterhouse owner, not the workers. In her blogpost entitled "The Crime of Indifference," Debra Roppolo writes, "But when those slaughterhouse workers chose to kill injured piglets rather than let them go to sanctuary, it broke something in the spirit of every animal-lover I know. *How could they?*"

Sometimes it hurts deeply to care. Veganism is one way we focus our care for animals; we choose food and clothing that do not support the slaughterhouse. Caring is vital to our activism and even to the most basic theory of veganism.

Why don't we hear more about caring in all the conversations about veganism? One reason is that besides engaging in disease shaming, our culture also enacts what we could call *care shaming*. Feeling compassion for animals is cast as emotional, and the emotional is cast as childish (animal activists being told to "grow up") or feminine (calling men who care about animals "sissy," or saying, "Man up!"). In addition, the vegan movement came of age in the midst of discussions about animal *rights* and animal *liberation*. Animal rights philosophy argues that animals have the right not to be used, not to be exploited by humans. Animal liberation philosophy says we need to consider the animals' *interests*, rather than asserting their rights. But both of these theories are flawed. Animal rights and animal liberation both view humans as autonomous, separate, and independent beings. This is not consistent with how we interact with one another in the world.

Understanding Our Interdependency
The theories of rights and liberation ignore the fact that we're not truly independent at all. We live in community and are actually *interdependent.*

What do we mean by this? Animal activist and artist Sunaura Taylor suggests that humans (and often nonhumans) are, "interdependent beings who care and rely on each other." That is, we are entangled together in life, and care will always be an aspect of this entanglement. This requires that we recognize that being dependent and vulnerable are not inherently bad.

In her book *Beasts of Burden: Animal and Disability Liberation*, Taylor writes,

> As human beings our dependence on each other is actually a minuscule amount of our overall dependence. We are massively dependent on other animals and of course on our environments in ways that are impossible for us to really even fathom. Other animals are dependent on their communities, habitats, and ecosystems. None of us is actually independent. The whole planet is interdependent.

We begin life dependent on others, and to some degree we remain dependent on others throughout our lives, just as others remain dependent on us. Eva Feder Kittay is a professor of philosophy at Stony Brook University where her work focuses in part on disability studies. She points out that disability is often just one variety of a dependency that we've all experienced at some point. She notes that the care of a disabled person who requires assistance is just one type of care that we give to people. Dr. Kittay writes, "I believe that we as a society have to end our fear and loathing of dependency. We need to see our dependency and our vulnerability to dependency as species-typical."

In other words, the idea that we are autonomous, which lies at the heart of animal rights and animal liberation, is a fiction.

Considerable personal benefits arise when we take the stigma out of dependency and recognize how dependent we are on others. Doing so allows us to acknowledge not just the problem with disease shaming and care shaming, but importantly our dependence on animals. We are invited to imagine different relationships, beginning with recognizing the role of animals in our lives.

A major tenet of Buddhism is interdependence. According to the Buddhist understanding of interdependence, all that exists, living beings included, is here because of and in relation to all else that exists. We are codependent with everyone and everything else in the universe.

But when we view dependency as "bad" and also view animals as dependent beings, separate from humans and from one another, it is easy to see animals as being here for our convenience. It becomes enticing and feels natural to exploit them.

Philosopher, ecofeminist, and critical animal studies scholar Lori Gruen has pioneered the idea of *entanglement* in her book *Entangled Empathy*. Through empathy, we have a means for caring for others, including other animals. She writes:

Being in ethical relations involves, in part, being able to understand and respond to another's needs, interests, desires, vulnerabilities, hopes, perspectives, etc. not simply by positing, from one's own point of view, what they might or should be but by working to try to grasp them from the perspective of the other.

A Vegan Ethic of Care

This entangled empathy points to an *ethic of care*. When our interdependence is a given, our caring is both an ethical responsibility and a gift.

Why hasn't the ethic of care been central to vegan activism? One reason might be that our culture disdains emotions and reduces "care" to an emotional state rather than seeing it as a vital part of our idea of justice. Also, the idea of an ethic of care comes from feminist theory, and we still live in a society in which women's contributions to philosophical theory are not given much attention or taken seriously. Still, this ethic of care is critical for us as activists in thinking about how to respond to our own or others' illnesses.

What does a vegan ethic of care look like? We suggest that it has four components: attention/holding space; activism; acceptance of grief; and acknowledging interdependence.

(1) *Attention and holding space*

The twentieth-century French mystic Simone Weil wrote: "The love of our neighbor in all its fullness simply means being able to say, 'What are you going through?'" and that we must be willing to listen for an answer. We vegans believe other animals count as our neighbors, and we believe that the question "What are you going through?" is being answered by animals all the time. With a vegan ethic of care we would bring that same attention and question to our fellow vegans who might be suffering. And we would pause to hear their answer, rather than assuming an answer. It is ironic that many vegans bring their attention and care so easily to animals, but need to be reminded to extend that care and attention to the people in their lives as well.

By asking, "What are you going through?" we offer kind attention, not judgment or stigmatization. We provide specific and very practical suggestions for caregiving in the next chapter, but want to suggest here the concept and practice of "holding space" for another. This holding space could be with someone who is ill, with the caregivers of someone who is ill, or with anyone who mourns.

In her article "What It Really Means to Hold Space for Someone," Heather Plett describes the concept this way:

> It means that we are willing to walk alongside another person in whatever journey they're on without judging them, making them feel inadequate, trying to fix them, or trying to impact the outcome. When we hold space for other people, we open our hearts, offer unconditional support, and let go of judgment and control.

(2) ACTIVISM

Many aspects of animal activism represent the enacting of the vegan ethic of care: participating in open rescues; working at shelters; fostering animals; adopting homeless animals; protesting against slaughterhouses, rodeos, fishing, hunting, and vivisection; educating others about animal exploitation and raising awareness through events; and letter-writing. Serving delicious vegan food is a form of activism, too. As a part of a vegan ethic of care, the activism needs to be inclusive of all vegans, not just those who adhere to some cultural notion of what a "good" vegan looks like.

(3) ACCEPTANCE OF GRIEF

For vegans, mourning is a given in a culture that continues to kill animals. Because we care, we often experience grief. But we have discovered that grief is nothing to fear. Caring is a gift. We won't privatize it or be ashamed of it (see chapter 6 on "Mourning").

A vegan ethic of care acknowledges that the powerful emotions that accompany our awareness of what is happening to animals are legitimate. So is our activism. We can affirm these emotions and face them without fear when we view veganism within the context of an ethic of care. Doing so equips us not to let these emotions overwhelm us. We can also use attention to understand the systemic forces that have deemed animals' lives immaterial. This ethic of care helps us resist feeling discouraged when other people don't care.

TIPS FOR HOLDING SPACE

1. Give people permission to trust their own intuition and wisdom.
2. Give people only as much information as they ask for and can handle so you don't overwhelm them or make them feel incompetent.
3. Don't take away their decision-making power.
4. Keep your own ego out of it.
5. Make them feel safe enough to fail by withholding shame and judgment.
6. Give guidance and help with humility and thoughtfulness, and know when to withhold guidance.
7. Create a safe container for complex emotions, fear, trauma, and so forth, if someone wishes to express them. ✎

(4) Acknowledging Interdependence

This is especially important in caregiving. Someone ill or dying may fear loss of autonomy as their activities of daily living (ADLs) become more challenging. ADLs include toileting, bathing, dressing, feeding oneself. In our culture, ADLs equal autonomy. But when we recognize that none of us is truly autonomous, we can help others become more comfortable with their needs. They are simply one more example of our interdependency. Especially when caregiving for animal activists, we need to help them see that those who care for animals may also be recipients of care. If we are caregivers, we need to learn how to ask for help from others and not believe we must do it all ourselves.

Caregiving, like the ethics of care itself, is always responding to a specific situation: the person's needs that day when they might be feeling well are different from their needs another day, when a blood transfusion has worn off, or they are more confused, or tired. Their needs in January might be different from their needs in June. Illness is not a static event between the loved one and a caregiver, and both recovery and dying can take time.

A vegan ethic of care provides a framework for our compassion, whether for other animals or people. It can be transformative for the vegan community because it offers us a method for supporting others who are ill or dying and for seeing ourselves as both potential caregivers *and* care receivers.

When Someone You Love Is
Seriously Ill or Dying

Susan Sontag famously opens her 1978 book, *Illness as Metaphor*, with the following:

> Illness is the night-side of life, a more onerous citizenship. Everyone who is born holds dual citizenship in the Kingdom of the Well and the Kingdom of the Sick. Although we all prefer to use only the good passport, sooner or later, each of us is obliged, at least for a spell, to identify ourselves as citizens of that other place.

The challenge for those of us holding the "good" passport is how we move in the Kingdom of the Sick—and, more importantly, how we help. As with any travel, there are etiquette *do's* and *don'ts*. It may be obvious, but let's state explicitly the reason why these etiquette tips are necessary: *The care of the person takes precedence.*

Don't . . .

1. Shame or blame. Don't ask, "What did you do wrong?" This is an inappropriate (and insulting) way to frame

serious illnesses. It is blaming the victim. If we see the person as failing at something, we may be seeking reassurance that it won't happen to us. Though we're not alone in seeing illness as a failure, this approach has additional repercussions for a person who is a vegan. Our need to be reassured that veganism didn't fail may cause the person to feel a failure as a vegan. We fail to care for that person when we see them as symbols of something— in this case, failed veganism—rather than for her or his own embodied reality. Illness is not shameful. Ill bodies are not shameful. Death is not shameful. Dying bodies are not shameful. Illness and dying are natural and certain, regardless of our diets or other lifestyle choices.

2. Say to a vegan, "You must have cheated." That is another way of blaming the victim, vegan style. If the person failed, our thinking goes, then veganism didn't.

3. Say, "But you're vegan." Again, this view of veganism as all-powerful protection is unrealistic.

4. Make their illness about you. If you reach out to them or their caregivers and no one gets back to you, it's not personal. They are in the middle of responding to illness.

5. Take it personally if you are not allowed to visit the person. The person may not be comfortable with changes in their body. They may want to be attended to by specific people, like family or people with health care expertise. They may feel a responsibility to entertain visitors and use up limited energy needed for essential care. They may need time to develop a care plan. They may be introverted. They may wish for time to interact with and reassure their companion animals. But whatever the reason, it's none of our business why we can't see them, and the refusal is not about us.

6. Stop by without an invitation unless explicitly told it is OK.

7. Assume you can be the exception to any rule or guideline, by saying, "Oh, they'd make an exception for me." It's not fair to place this burden on the ill person. Whether it's true in some ideal world of your friendship doesn't matter. They are not living in that ideal world.

8. Ask them, "Do you think you'll still be alive by . . . ?" This is immensely hurtful.

9. Ask them to become your guru (or travel guide) since they are now a resident of the Kingdom of the Sick. Their role is not to educate you or reassure you or care for you and your pain at their illness; they are not obligated to have developed beautiful insights about their situation to pass on to you.

10. Visit because you need closure, because you want to hear something profound that you think will reconcile you to their dying. This is unfair and cruel. It is this individual's life. Let them live it their way up to their death. Their optimism may be the most significant frame of mind they have in the face of pain and loss. Closure may not be as necessary to them as it is to you. They may be using their energy to think about living, not dying. Their hope of living carries value to them. Don't smother it with your need for closure.

11. Demand information.

12. Make them responsible for your feelings.

13. Impose your needs on them. (See all of the above!)

14. Say, "Everything is for a purpose."

15. Say you know someone who had it and got better.

16. Use social media as an avenue for closure. For instance, don't eulogize them before their death. Don't post things on Facebook about the person in the third person. Don't make a video about the person and post to social media without permission.

17. Become a chore for the caregivers.
18. Talk *at* the person.
19. Talk *about* the person in front of the person, especially if you are conversing with their medical team or other caregivers.
20. Say, "If only. . . ."
21. Reduce complex issues of life and death to simplistic and supposed "remedies."
22. Give unasked-for advice. Something may have some anticancer properties, for instance, but this does not mean it can cure cancer.
23. Feel you have to solve the situation. Activists are used to having skills for solving situations. But don't bring the expectation that you can solve your loved one's illness to your interactions with that loved one.

With all these recommendations, we aren't trying to frighten you into believing that you'll be inept or inappropriate and so you shouldn't do anything. No, not by any means. But these *don'ts* indicate that, when we aren't thoughtful, when we respond with our own needs instead of the needs of the ill person, we may be hurtful unintentionally.

When he was living with a terminal diagnosis, Tom Lubbock, the art critic for the UK *Independent* newspaper, described three annoying sympathizers:

1. Those who come only wanting to have their minds put at rest.
2. Those who know someone who had exactly what you've got, and she's absolutely fine now.
3. Those who want you to know they realize just how awful it is for you—and with the little one! [They had a very young child.]

None of these sympathizers responded with attentiveness, open to hearing what he was going through, but offered their own opinions instead.

As the brother of a woman who suffered from sarcoma-tissue cancer for fifteen years, Steven Thrasher experienced many tiresome and relentless advice-givers. In an article for the *Guardian* published after his sister's death, he wrote, "Don't tell cancer patients what they could be doing to cure themselves." He suggests it is our anxiety about our own mortality that causes us to advise cancer patients, even though we have not been invited to give our advice. He characterizes it as a "sneaky and harmful way of dealing with your own fear of death."

We know it is not only vegans who do this. Religious people advise prayer. Laws-of-attraction folks propose adopting a positive attitude. Juice fasters? They advise juice-fasting. As vegans, we are often advice-givers. Our bumper stickers, T-shirts, and other public statements embed the advice GO VEGAN. But don't start in now with advice.

Thrasher describes the situation this way:

> My sister was a PhD and a licensed psychologist, and she fought hard as a black woman to establish her place in the medical profession. Why would people look at her and think, Well, in all these years of facing death, as a doctor consulting other doctors, she is probably so lacking in intellectual curiosity—or she is such a stooge of Big Pharma—that I bet she hasn't considered this advice I read in a magazine?!

Even if our advice comes from our lives and not a magazine, still, we should not give it unless explicitly asked for it.

Thrasher identifies several problems with advice-giving:

- It's condescending. It assumes the individual and their care team don't know what they are doing.
- It's an inadequate substitute for the practical help that is actually needed.
- Giving advice "blames the sick person for your discomfort with their reality and shifts any accountability you feel back on them."
- It further separates the sick person from community by concluding they were in control and failed to prevent or heal themselves of the illness.

Here's a sound bite for guidance: "Not your disease; not your opinion."

Do . . .

1. Learn to be comfortable with your discomfort about what is happening to the person you love, or learn to push past the discomfort to actual engagement with the actual person.
2. Accept if the person doesn't want to see you that it's nothing personal.
3. Protect their privacy.
4. Ask permission before you do something that has a widespread effect or that disseminates information that is at all sensitive or has the potential to reveal personal information to others. For instance, do ask if it is okay to create a GoFundMe campaign, a Caring Bridge link, or Facebook post.
5. Accept whatever role you are invited to have, and understand that that is the most essential thing you can do, even if it does not bring direct contact with the person who is ill. (See pages 49–51 for more on this.)

6. Be mindful of the physical limits on the person who is ill. Your visit could contribute to your loved one's exhaustion.

7. Accept that there might be nothing you can do. That is the *something* you have to do: nothing.

8. Ask them what they want.

9. Keep the commitments for caregiving that you make. Even if you think the task you have agreed to do seems inconsequential, your "yes" has been factored into a care schedule.

10. Be an active listener and keep your judgment and needs out of it. Offer comfort and support. You can say, "I'm sorry this has happened." Comfort is not advice. Comfort is not opinion. Comfort is not what you feel.

11. Offer practical help.

12. Sit with them, if this is welcomed. Accept silence and know that presence is a gift in itself. Or read to them, if that is appropriate.

13. If you have always said, "I love you," continue to say it.

Understand that you may feel anxious in providing direct care. If you aren't a trained health care professional you may worry about "doing the wrong thing." The week Carol's mother was dying, she noticed this anxiety in herself. But she also learned through caregiving that notions of perfectionism had no place at the sickbed. We try to do the best we can, that is all we can do; but the trying and the caring become powerful antidotes to anxiety and perfectionism. When we were babies, our parents often didn't know how to care for us either. They showed up (well, most of them) and did the best they could, learning as they went. Remember that care is imperfect and this fact may help you when you offer it.

You Get over It

Awareness of our dying, whether sped up by a terminal diagnosis or not, confronts us with the limits of our bodies. So does caregiving. When Carol arrived to help care for her mother, who had been suffering from Alzheimer's for many years but now had an undiagnosed illness that had severely weakened her, Carol found that at first it was difficult to change her mother's adult diapers. She confided this to a friend, who had been caring for her own father who also had dementia for several years. Carol said, "I'm squeamish." Her friend said lightly, "You get over it." She was right; you do. Another time, caring for her elderly mother-in-law whose leg had recently been amputated, Carol was called into the room. As she approached the commode to empty it, her mother-in-law told her, "I did both." Carol wanted to be compassionate but she did not want to deal with bodily fluids. Then she realized compassion *is* dealing with bodily fluids. Compassion is accepting and loving the body. ✎

The Ring Theory

After clinical psychologist Susan Silk developed breast cancer, she heard many inappropriate comments. She and law-school professor Barry Goldman wrote an op-ed for the *Los Angeles Times* entitled, "How Not to Say the Wrong Thing." They devised what they call "The Ring Theory" of kvetching. Start by drawing a small circle in the middle of a page. Inside this circle goes the name of the person who is seriously ill or dying, the person with the "bad passport." Then draw a larger circle around the first one. In this circle, put the name(s) of the person(s) closest to the individual who is sick or dying. These individuals, the next closest to the individual in the center, may be parents, children, intimate friends (versus less-intimate friends).

Repeat the process of drawing circles around the inner circles as many times as needed to account for relations, friends, activists, coworkers, and so forth. For instance, there may be different levels of intimacy among animal activists, and some may be in an inner ring around the center circle and some may be in an outer ring.

The rule that Silk and Goldman developed is that the person in the center ring "can say anything she wants to anyone, anywhere. She can kvetch and complain and whine and moan and curse the heavens and say, 'Life is unfair!' and 'Why me?'" They call this "kvetching out."

Everyone else can also "kvetch out." That is, they can complain and share their feelings with others, but only to those who are in larger rings. When talking to someone in circles closer to the center, the goal is to help and listen.

The rule is: "Comfort in, dump out." Wherever you are in the circle, you know you aren't the one in the center with the bad passport. So, "comfort in, dump [or kvetch] out."

Now that we've cleared the air a bit on some of the problematic responses to serious illness, let's explore more closely the two kingdoms of the well and the sick. First, we don't think it should actually be called a "bad passport." *Bad* is a judgmental word. The situation requires a suspension of judgment. Instead, the sick person has been given a new passport that changes their travel—both the time that remains to them and where their journey will take them. What do they need from us?

Individuals who become caregivers find themselves residing in a kingdom that is not the Kingdom of the Well. Caregiving is its own world, disrupting the borders of the world caregivers thought they resided in. Different laws take precedence in this world:

- The law of **gravity** is magnified. Falls happen more frequently and not just to the person who is ill. Research shows that caregivers are more prone to falling than the average person—perhaps an expression of the trauma associated with caregiving.
- The law of **inertia**. A body at rest will stay at rest, especially after a fall. This law is often experienced by a caregiver, for instance attempting to lift someone who has fallen out of a wheelchair. A body in motion will stay in motion, especially the body of the caregiver, who, when finally having an opportunity to rest, cannot calm down heart or mind sufficiently to fall asleep.
- The law of **time**. Sometimes, everything is very urgent and minutes matter. Sometimes, we sit in the hospital for hours waiting for a doctor's consultation. Sometimes, we realize simply sitting with someone is all that matters. Clocks rise and fall in importance.
- The law of **allegiances**. The caregiver's primary concern is the person in the center of the ring.

Which Circle Are You In?

Going back to our ring theory, determining your role in relationship to the person who is ill means figuring out which circle you're in.

We suggest that some grouping of those in the immediate circle surrounding the center circle will probably become a part of the *Care Team*: close family members and/or intimate friends.

RESPONSIBILITIES OF THE CARE TEAM

1. Find out what the person who is ill wants.
2. Enforce what they want.
3. Interface with the Care Support Team (see below).
4. Accompany the individual to medical appointments,

be an advocate for their wishes, ask about medications, and take notes. There are times when it is appropriate to question the plan of care being developed, and to push and find alternative solutions.

5. At least one or more individuals on the care team should be on the person's HIPAA. Federal rules regarding the disclosure of health information were enacted with the adoption of the Health Insurance Portability and Accountability Act (HIPAA). Unless the patient has signed a HIPAA form allowing for disclosure, medical professionals cannot discuss the patient's health, prognosis, or medical needs with another family member or friend.

COPING AND CARING: 10 TIPS

Carol's friend Pamela was "the total care partner" of her husband Bill after he developed an atypical form of Parkinsonism, Progressive Supranuclear Palsy (PSP). After several years of intense and demanding caregiving, Pamela gave a TEDX talk about hers and Bill's life together. "He is not 'fighting' or 'battling' his disease," she said.

It is untreatable. He is making the best possible life with PSP. Several times a day, his reply to me is, "That's lucky!" As our sons say, "Dad is showing us how to make the best of a bad situation."

Bill has shown me and everyone that loves him dignity in extreme illness. There is his grace with patience and acceptance. It sometimes takes him five minutes to pry his eyes open. He has faith and gentleness. I have never heard one complaint (about anything!). His wisdom is in knowing what is truly important. He has done this all with bottomless love. He has taught us to love what is.

I am always reading and searching for tips on how to cope and care. Each case is as individual as a fingerprint. From our experiences, here are my own top ten tips:

1. What you do repeatedly has great power to change you, for better or worse. This is worth repeating.
2. Laugh . . . with each other, at movies, with friends; whatever it takes, just laugh.
3. Get help, paid or unpaid. It is impossible alone. Self-pity sucks.
4. Exercise helps with depression. I love yoga and swimming. We both chair dance.
5. Music lifts spirits. Keep the music coming.
6. Remember, you can only choose your reactions, not the situations.
7. Flow and pause; breathe. As you move from task to task; flow, pause, breathe.
8. How I want to act is with kindness and courage. Remind yourself, when you hate everything.
9. Get out of the four walls, every day if possible. Try to think of something out of the rut.
10. Keep changing the solutions as the problems change.

The Care Team needs support, too, since they may become overwhelmed giving direct care to the ill person. That support comes from those in the next circle, the *Care Support Team*. By supporting the Care Team, you are also supporting the loved one in the center of the circle. It may feel like indirect support, but it is not. Anything that frees the caregivers' energy and time to attend to the ill person directly touches that person. There is no hierarchy of who is more important and what tasks are more necessary; there are needs and there is the question, "Who can meet them?" The desire to help is always weighed against the loved one's needs for help and who they want to have helping.

Responsibilities of the Care Support Team will vary depending on the circumstances. But we can think of a number of tasks that are likely to be necessary when the person who is ill is a vegan or when the caretakers are vegan. For example, many vegans and animal activists have adopted animals, and this often includes animals with special needs. And whereas neighbors and families may be eager to help with meals, they may not have the skills or knowledge for providing nourishing vegan food as well as vegan comfort food and treats.

POTENTIAL RESPONSIBILITIES OF THE CARE SUPPORT TEAM
1. Care for animals in the home.
    - Walk dogs; check on them on long days when the loved one is at the hospital for tests, checkups, chemo, or radiation.
    - Provide medical care for animals with special needs. Realistically understand what is needed.
    - Be on the kitty-litter cleanup team.
    - Be on "vet duty" if a companion animal needs a medical appointment.
2. Care for animals outside the home.
    - If the person who is ill regularly feeds birds or a colony of community cats, you might step in and help with that.

Marion Couts, the widow of Tom Lubbock who was dying of a brain tumor and whom we quoted earlier in this chapter, wrote a remarkable memoir, *The Iceberg*. In it, she identifies her three jobs as a caregiver:

1. Not to let Tom be destroyed before his death but to help him live it fully in his own way with all his power.
2. Not to let Ev [their young son] be destroyed by Tom's death but to help him live it fully in his own way with all his power.
3. Not to let myself be destroyed. See 1 and 2.

That's it. ✎

3. Be on the food team. Even if the person who is ill has little appetite or has special food needs, such as blended foods, the care team members still need to eat. Arrange for food to be delivered through a sign-up of others who care and wish to do something. Remind the ones who signed up of their day and time. Instruct them on how to deliver the food.
   - Be on grocery duty—shopping for food and delivering it.
   - Be a person who makes and delivers meals.
   - Prepare food in small containers for freezing for the caregivers so there is always something available.
   - Deliver vegan food to the hospital for the caregivers during an operation and when 24-hour care is being provided at the hospital. (Who doesn't know, at this point, how wretched and un-vegan most hospital food is?)
4. Maintain communication on behalf of the care team.
   - Maintain a phone tree, so that when a need exists (more food, transportation to a medical appointment, and so on), individuals are already identified who might be available.

- Provide updates, with the explicit permission of the loved one (through Caring Bridge, emails, or Facebook).
- Interface with those who want to visit. Set limits: for instance, "short visits" may be welcome, but boundaries must be explicit.
- Suggest other tangible ways of remaining present to the person: cards, pictures, notes, flowers. This is a time for snail mail.

5. Support the care team.
   - Be an active listener.
   - Arrange for a massage if that's something the caregiver would enjoy.
   - Refrain from asking them to meet your needs.

6. Research vegan resources for the ill person.
   - Examine the menus at the hospital, assisted-living facility, or hospice, and work to get vegan options for the person. Look for inappropriate ingredients and educate without being bossy or causing ill feelings toward the sick person. Assume a lack of understanding by medical professionals about what a vegan is, so that you don't use up your time or theirs with frustration. Be kind. "No, yogurt from cow's milk is not vegan. But these kinds of yogurt would work." "No, gluten-free and vegan are not the same thing. Here's a list of what vegans don't eat."
   - Investigate vegan alternatives for medications being prescribed. This research is done, of course, with the permission of the person who is ill. But vegans generally wish to avoid medication that contains animal products. When Lisa Shapiro, a beloved vegan activist, was dying, the doctors wanted her to take a medication from pigs to clear out her veins; research revealed that a vegan alternative existed.

7. Help with household chores.
   - Wash sheets, clean out the refrigerator.
   - Maintain cars.
   - Mow the lawn, weed the garden, or shovel snow.
   - Help retrofit the home or apartment with railing grips, ramps, and other aids to stability. Needless to say, this is a task for someone with some carpentry skills.
8. Help with accounting tasks.
   - Interface and advocate with insurance companies.
   - Manage bills and follow up on billings that may have been incorrect.

Each person is going to have separate needs influenced by their own personality and where in the Kingdom of the Sick the passport has permitted them entry. What is vital is to personalize the caring response for each individual. Caregiving is situational. In addition, often one group of people actually fulfills the tasks we've separated into teams. (We aren't trying to be exhaustive in this section, but want to highlight essential issues and specifically vegan-related issues. For a discussion of the concerns of caregivers see the chapter on "Veganism and Caregiving" in *Never Too Late to Go Vegan*.)

Finally, it may be necessary as a caregiver to engage in an advanced planning guide with the person who is ill. Different states have different requirements for Do Not Resuscitate (DNR) forms and Medical Proxy forms; however, we have found *Five Wishes* a very helpful instrument for assuring yourself and the care receiver that you know what they want. This tool can clarify who will be making the critical medical decisions for the person who is ill and what kind of treatment the person wants, as well as other personal decisions about care. We discuss *Five Wishes* and other end-of-life issues in much more depth in chapters 5 and 7.

A year and a half after her husband was diagnosed with a brain tumor, Marion Couts wrote:

> Maybe all that can be spoken by me at this time is not about happiness or unhappiness, or optimism or competition, but just that we are all still here. To be still here is all there is. This page marks our presence. In the light of that fact either I do not despair or I suppress despair. I cannot tell which. Plenty of time to work that out later.

We are still here: That is our witness and reassurance to someone who is ill or dying.

Part 3

A Vegan's Guide
to Death and Dying

When You Have a Terminal Illness

"WE ALL LIVE WITH A DEATH SENTENCE," PRONOUNCED WALTER White in television's *Breaking Bad*. Through a terminal illness, some of us learn its approximate date; others of us will never know it. French writer Maurice Blanchot suggests we can never know—or write about—the disaster that is our death. Well, what he writes is more complicated than this, but for our purposes let us say: We may know our dying, but we cannot know our own death. Tom Lubbock lived for two years after the diagnosis of a malignant brain tumor. One month after the diagnosis, he wrote: "The living thing strives to live. The living thing has a stop. . . . The shape of the creature is the pressure of life against the limit of death."

No matter what we have read or come to believe, we vegans don't escape the death sentence. We, too, will die. We, too, live with the pressure of life against the limit of death. It's something our culture wants to ignore, though.

Katherine Russell Rich, a journalist with breast cancer, was called into her editor's room for a staff appraisal.

> "Sit down," he said gruffly. He didn't look like a man who wanted to talk. He looked like a man who was

under orders from Personnel to deliver the corporate report cards.

"I don't know what to say to you," he began. "I can't review your work. You haven't done much this year. I haven't wanted to give you things to do. Partly for humanitarian reasons. But partly because I wanted to be sure that they got done."

But they would have, I assured him. And you can begin now, I said.

Smiling, he said he would. "You know," he chortled. "I really felt bad for you. No one here wanted anything to do with you because you reminded them they could die."

Living with a Death Sentence

Learning that you have a terminal illness is likely to bring on a range of emotions—fear, anger, sadness, helplessness, a sense of disbelief. There is no right way to feel and no right way to deal with the knowledge of your diagnosis. Studies of people who have terminal illnesses can give us some insight on helpful strategies. A 2005 study conducted by a group of Australian doctors and psychologists found that coping strategies for those with a terminal illness included trying to maintain a sense of normality and routine, doing enjoyable things, and remembering that life doesn't stop with a terminal diagnosis.

Eulogizing Lisa Shapiro who died from cancer in 2015, her friend Paul Shapiro wrote about some of their last conversations:

Just a few weeks before her death, I was talking with Lisa by phone while she lay on what she very clearly knew was likely to be her deathbed. I listened to her struggles and hopes, and shared my thoughts on where our movement is headed. She told me many things, but what struck me most was that, even in her compromised state, she never stopped advocating for animals.

"My eyesight's not good due to my pain meds," Lisa would tell her friends who aren't part of the animal movement, as a means of getting them to read her articles about vegan eating and animal protection. She casually quipped to me, "I'm dying—what are they gonna do, say no?" And it worked. Some of them told her they were already starting to eat less meat because of those readings.

Lisa knew she was dying, but she also knew that her life wasn't over. She was still finding ways to do what was meaningful to her, which was to have an impact for animals.

Acknowledging that you are going to die allows you to begin planning how you will use the rest of your life—whether it is measured in years or months or weeks. And how you spend that time will depend on your own resources and, of course, on what matters most to you. Maybe you'll choose to put time and energy toward making a difference for animals. It might be volunteering at the animal shelter, protesting the circus, writing letters to the editor, or making vegan cooking videos for Facebook. You may find ways to sneak a little activism into your daily routine. You might even see that allowing others to bring you meals is a type of activism; at the very least, they will learn that mashed potatoes are just as good with soymilk as cow's milk, and that vegan chili is easier to make and just as tasty as the meaty kind.

It's also possible that at this stage of your life you want to turn your focus to the more personal things that bring you comfort— more time with family and friends and pets, more time engaged in spiritual activities. Or maybe you want to travel to favorite places or somewhere new that you've always wanted to go.

You might want to look to the future, writing letters or making videos for those you love, especially for young children. Maybe you'll even throw a party, asking friends and family to celebrate your life with you, sharing memories and stories.

How you spend your time is always a personal decision and that doesn't change with the knowledge that time is limited. Some people want to do and see all of the things they postponed when they thought they had all the time in the world. Others are comforted by a sense of routine and don't want to change a thing. Either approach allows you to live life to its fullest, however you define it. As one of Lisa Shapiro's caregivers told us, "You still want to find what has been feeding you, and let it keep feeding you even when you are dying."

Communicating with Others

People are not comfortable with death—it's one of the reasons we wrote this book after all—and many feel especially uncomfortable about being around someone who is dying. They don't know what to say or how to act. And they would just as soon avoid any reminder of their own mortality.

Some might be reluctant to visit and, as sad as that is, it's not about their lack of concern for you. Likewise, people may wish to visit at times when you don't want company or prefer to have the company of just a few people of your choosing.

In either case, you might find other ways to stay in touch and also to let people know what you need. The free Caring Bridge website gives you the opportunity to share news with all of your loved ones in one private, safe place. It's also an opportunity to ask for help and to let others coordinate that help. You can decide who will read the entries and can keep your page private, by invitation only, or make it public.

Whether you are maintaining contact with family and friends in person or by written communication or through the

Internet, you'll need to tell them what you need, and just as importantly, what you don't need. No matter how close your family and friends are to you, they can't know what you are feeling and what you are going through. They can't know whether their stories and advice about treatments and hope are helpful or hurtful.

Let people know that you've done your research and are comfortable with the treatment you've chosen or with your decision to discontinue treatment. You can tell loved ones that further discussion or advice about this will only distract you from the business at hand, which is living the rest of your life in the way that brings you happiness and feels right to you.

Your Care
Information is a very useful strategy for coping with major life events. It can be helpful to know as much as possible about your disease and any treatment options so that you can be an active participant in all decisions about treatment and care.

If you have chosen care in a hospice facility, you'll want to talk with them about your vegan diet. You may want to arrange for someone else to bring you food if you can't be at home and if the facility is not familiar with vegan diets. Even if friends or family are caring for you at home, you may need to provide information about what you eat, and point them to your stash of vegan cookbooks.

Although still in the minority, a growing number of hospitals and hospice facilities allow visits from pets. Many also have therapy-dog programs. It's not nearly as comforting as seeing your own furry loved one, but a visit from any animal can be uplifting and cheering. Talk to hospice care providers about your nonhuman family members and how much they mean to you, and ask for arrangements that will allow you to continue to see them.

FIVE WISHES

Five Wishes has been dubbed "a living will with a heart and soul." As a will, this document addresses legal issues regarding end-of-life care. However, what makes *Five Wishes* unique is that it also allows you to address personal, spiritual, and emotional wishes as they pertain to your care.

Wishes one and two are the legal parts of the document:

WISH 1: THE PERSON I WANT TO MAKE CARE DECISIONS FOR ME WHEN I CAN'T

This section is an assignment of a health care power of attorney, the person who will make medical decisions on your behalf if you are no longer able to do so.

WISH 2: THE KIND OF MEDICAL TREATMENT I WANT OR DON'T WANT

This is the living will portion of the document. It allows you to define what type of life-support treatment you want or don't want.

Wishes 3 through 5 provide an opportunity to be specific about your personal needs and desires, and to describe the kind of care you want. These are the wishes that make the document unique since they address comfort care, spirituality, forgiveness, and final wishes.

WISH 3: HOW COMFORTABLE I WANT TO BE

This section addresses matters of comfort care, including what type of pain management you would like and instructions about bathing and personal grooming.

WISH 4: HOW I WANT PEOPLE TO TREAT ME

Here, you can specify any number of things that might bring you comfort—whether or not you would like people to pray for you, play your favorite music, or read favorite poems. You can specify which people you want with you and whether you want your pets nearby.

WISH 5: WHAT I WANT MY LOVED ONES TO KNOW

This section deals with matters of forgiveness, how you wish to be remembered, and final wishes regarding any memorials.

Because the document is so personal, there are opportunities for you, as a vegan, to make some specific wishes known. For example, you might want to specify the types of vegan products you'd like used in your personal care. You can ask that your commitment to animals be remembered in a memorial service or celebration of your life. You can specify a charity to receive contributions in your memory. You can ask that food served at a memorial is vegan.

When signed and witnessed by two people, *Five Wishes* is a fully legal document. According to the American Bar Association Commission on Law and Aging, it currently meets the legal requirements for an advance directive in 42 states and the District of Columbia. *Five Wishes* can be used in the remaining states with additional documentation.

If you already have a living will or a durable power or attorney, *Five Wishes* can replace those documents if you destroy the original and write "revoked" on the copies. You can download the *Five Wishes* document from the Last Visit website or from Aging with Dignity.

Coping with Guilt and Shame

Despite the inevitability of death for every living being, for vegans there can be a sense of guilt and shame around dying—and maybe some anger over a sense of unfairness. You've lived a life of compassion and advocacy for animals. You've treated your body well, especially compared to how the average person eats. You might feel that your body has failed you, or you've failed your body.

The embarrassment that some vegans feel when they are sick is magnified when the sickness turns into something life threatening.

On the other hand, to meat eaters your illness becomes proof of the fallibility, if not the failure, of veganism.

A vegan activist who had breast cancer worried that if people knew she had been vegan for thirty years and she had breast cancer at fifty then they would not go vegan. Despite the fact that she could have had a genetic marker for breast cancer, or that environmental factors could have caused her cancer, she was concerned that after touting veganism for all those years her illness would be "bad" for veganism. In fact, she encountered some insensitive meat eaters. At least one said, "If this is what happens when you go vegan, then I don't want to go vegan."

Sometimes it seems that society revels in the news that a vegan is sick. In May 2016, the same week that vegan climber Kuntal Joisher made it to the top of Mount Everest, another vegan, Maria Strydom, died on her way to the summit. Her death was trumpeted, almost gleefully, by some news outlets and mocked by others, because one of her goals had been to prove that vegans could do anything. Instead she had died. Joisher, on the other hand, who did in fact prove that vegans can do anything, barely got a mention in the news.

But someone else's illness is not about us as individuals or as vegans. And no matter what we might believe if we are the ones who are ill, it is not about *our* veganism.

We know how to reduce risk for disease, not how to prevent it. In fact, even if your lifestyle was not particularly healthy, it doesn't mean you know why you got sick. People who have the healthiest possible habits according to current knowledge can still develop chronic diseases. More and more people are being diagnosed with lung cancer who never smoked cigarettes. As we age, more and more of us will be dying from all kinds of illnesses, regardless of how well we cared for ourselves. Compassion for ourselves and for others, who are ill or dying, is the only appropriate action when we are faced with these challenges.

It's key to let go of questions about why you became ill and to recognize and accept that some things are truly beyond our control, even as vegans. When you do that, you can comfortably talk about your diagnosis with others, and ask for the help and comfort you need.

Vegans may also feel a sense of dilemma about medications. Even if you are no longer treating your illness, you will likely take advantage of pain medication to manage symptoms. Most of it comes from companies that test on animals. If you have advocated against vivisection and animal testing in the past, you may question whether it's right to take advantage of these drugs.

But we live in an imperfect world and those who coined the term *vegan* back in 1944 knew that. The Vegan Society in the UK holds that veganism is, "a way of living which seeks to exclude, as far as is possible and practicable, all forms of exploitation of, and cruelty to, animals for food, clothing or any other purpose."

They included the clause about "as far as is possible and practicable" because even many years ago they knew that it wasn't possible to avoid every single animal product a hundred percent of the time. It is certainly possible to eat a diet free of animal products, and it is easier than ever to avoid the use of fur, leather, silk, and wool. But it's not at all practical to avoid driving a car or walking on asphalt, which contains animal ingredients.

It's not practical to eliminate music from your life because some musical instruments contain glue or strings derived from animals. It's not practical to never use house paint because it may contain the milk protein casein.

It is also not practical to refuse medication that you need when no alternative exists. There are times when the only choice is a non-vegan choice. We work toward a world where there are alternatives to all products that involve animal use. But that world does not yet exist.

Terminal Illness, Veganism, and Hope

Facing death encourages most people to spend some time reflecting on their lives. This life review, looking back at your accomplishments and the experiences and relationships that have given you joy, can help you achieve a sense of meaning at the end of your life.

These kinds of reflections can also be a mixed bag, of course. Life, after all, is a messy sort of stew made up of good and bad decisions, joys and regrets. Buddhists say that life itself is composed of ten thousand joys and ten thousand sorrows. There are likely to be some things you can fix if you're so inclined—an expression of gratitude that you never adequately conveyed or an apology that you've always wanted to make.

For the most part, though, there isn't much to be gained by focusing on what you wish you had done or had not done. Instead, as vegans, we have every reason to celebrate a life well lived. When people talk about their biggest regrets, one of the most common is this: "I wish I'd had the courage to live a life true to myself, not the life others expected of me."

As vegans, we choose to do just that—to live according to our values of compassion, fairness, and justice. We do so in a world that is not especially accommodating to these beliefs when it comes to animals or a vegan lifestyle.

As vegans, we live values that engender hope. Although hope is generally thought of as an expectation of a good future, something that seems incompatible with a terminal illness, physician Sherwin Nuland, who wrote the book *How We Die*, defines it differently. He says that, "hope resides in the meaning of what our lives have been."

It doesn't matter if you went vegan twenty years ago or just last month. It doesn't matter if every choice you made was perfectly vegan or if you struggled with veganism and slipped up now and again. It doesn't matter if you were an activist or were simply living quietly according to your values. Simply by embracing the ethic of veganism, we live lives of meaning and purpose. It means that even at the end of our lives, we are living with hope.

⊰ 6 ⊱

Mourning

We live with so much grief: our grief for being finite and having limited bodies; our grief for those who have died; and, of course, our grief for animals.

In one sense, we vegans are in mourning all the time. When we consider the vast numbers of animals slaughtered intentionally just for food every year—ten billion land animals in the United States alone, and thousands of billions more from the oceans worldwide, as well as animals killed in experiments and for feathers and fur—our hearts break and we grieve.

We are living and working in the midst of huge losses that touch us deeply but go unrecognized by the rest of the world. This ongoing atrocity is one reason we need to care for ourselves with fierce compassion. It's one reason we wrote this book—to speak to the importance of a vegan community that expresses compassion and acceptance for all its members.

When vegans mourn as a community, we support one another in our ongoing grief. This is the type of mourning that binds us as a community. Another, of course, is that each of us experiences personal loss. This is the acute and intense grief that comes when a close, loved one dies. As Barbara J. King writes in *How Animals Grieve*, "When grief slams into a life, the background hum of daily routine vanishes."

We mourn not just the person who died, but the roles we played in their presence. Suddenly, and awfully, we are no longer a caregiver, a sister, a daughter, a friend. Our grief is compounded by disorientation. We find ourselves in a new world, a new role, and it is neither by our choice nor to our liking.

Grieving

It is very hard to grieve. We want grief to be taken away from us, lifted from us. But it is never that easy. Structurally, our culture does not really allow grieving at all. We allow one week if you lose a spouse, two weeks if you lose a child. Then you are supposed to be fully functional. In all forms of grief, we don't allow enough time. The message we hear is, "Finish grieving and get back to living."

In a culture saturated with the denial of death, how we grieve becomes a mostly private event, except for a funeral or memorial service. Grief can be isolating, and we cannot stress enough how comforting it can be to be among other people when your grief is raw and new and overwhelming. When your grief is new and raw, you might want to ask friends to visit, to listen as you share stories about your loved one, perhaps for an hour a day, or for one day each week. If someone can sleep over and keep you company for a few days at least, you will have a safety zone in which to express your loss and be heard and held in comfort. Patricia Kelley writes, "Perhaps the most valuable lesson about loss and grief is . . . when we are grieving there is immeasurable value in the gift of presence—someone who will keep us company in our grief."

Kelley's advice can be found in her practical guide to mourning, *Companion to Grief: Finding Consolation When Someone You Love Has Died*. Her excellent, commonsense advice comes from years as a nurse and educator in hospice care. She explains that "the task of grieving is learning to live without the person who died." Whereas this may feel impossible and unwanted at first, day by day, mourning your loss and expressing your grief will lead to a kind of peace with the new reality of the tremendous hole in your life. While acknowledging that you can never replace the loved one who is gone, you can make strides in time and in finding other ways to fill the roles that person played in your life.

Reassuringly, Kelley tells us,

> You may feel very sad, very angry, very lonely, and the feelings may be so strong that you feel them physically. Over time, these feelings may diminish in intensity and frequency. Rather than an excruciating pain of loneliness, you'll feel a milder ache. Rather than being furious that she died and left you, you'll feel regret. Rather than feeling abandoned as the only person left in the world, you're lonely for the special times you used to share.
>
> Sometimes it isn't the intensity of the pain that diminishes, but the frequency with which you feel it. The pain of losing the person you love may be as severe as ever, but you feel that pain less often.

Mourning Rituals

Grief is a universal response to loss, yet the way we grieve varies among cultures, and among people even in the same family. Anthropologist Kelli Swazey describes a tradition from Tana Toraja, Indonesia, in which a funeral is a raucous, days- to weeks-long ceremony involving an entire village. The deceased's body is cared for among their family until a fitting funeral can be arranged, sometimes months after the death. In her riveting TED talk, Swazey shows us a culture in which death is not the end but the beginning of a new relationship with the departed.

Each religion offers its own mourning rituals, and rituals can be helpful to give us something to do when we are overwhelmed with grief. If we have a religious tradition, rituals can also offer

OUR BODIES, OUR GRIEF

We do everything through our bodies; sometimes it is grief that reminds us of this. We do not have any disembodied experiences. When we grieve we are truly stricken and stripped. C. S. Lewis wrote: "No one ever told me that grief felt so like fear. I am not afraid, but the sensation is like being afraid. The same fluttering in the stomach, the same restlessness, the yawning. I keep on swallowing." Grief, Lewis reminds us, is agonizingly bodily: stomach flutters, yawning, swallowing—"like being mildly drunk, or concussed, faint nausea," "feelings, and feelings, and feelings."

Grief, according to Carol's friend and body therapist Martha Murphy Hall, is a "polyglot emotive experience." It is not one feeling, but a group of feelings that rotate— anger, depression, guilt, acceptance, anger, depression, guilt . . . feelings, feelings, feelings. When we mourn, we experience the physicality of grief. We know this because our bodies ache: the stomachache, the loss of appetite, sleeplessness.

Grief teaches us that we have bodies and it teaches us about our capacity to care. The more we have loved, or experienced ourselves as attached to another, the more we will grieve.

comfort, whether they encourage us to mourn in community, promise us that our loved ones live on in an afterlife or in a future life, or give us opportunities to talk about the deceased loved one. Rituals also help us come to accept the reality of what feels unreal, the sudden absence of someone we loved, and the feeling and desperate hope that maybe we are dreaming and will wake up from this disturbing new, ongoing nightmare.

Catholics hold a Mass when someone dies. Some Christians hold a wake, a way to spend time with the body of the deceased before burial, share memories, and comfort one another. Jewish mourning calls for sitting shiva, gathering in the home of the deceased for a week (*shiva* means "seven") to remember the deceased and support the family with food and company. (Many Jews today sit for less than a week.) There is a tradition that requires a prayer called Kaddish to be recited daily for eleven months when a parent dies. Muslim community members bring food to the grieving family for at least a few days after a funeral and burial. When a Muslim woman loses her husband, it is traditional to mourn for four months and ten days. This mourning period is called 'Iddah. Official mourning can last forty days or more, though some Muslims mourn for shorter periods of time.

Whether or not a memorial includes a religious component, many will provide an opportunity to share photos, stories, and declarations of love. It is an act of love and generosity to plan and conduct a memorial service. It can be thought of as the last gift you can give to your loved one. People frequently remark, "He would have loved this!" when the memorial is in the style or includes the music, art, or other passions the deceased used to enjoy. Including the deceased's favorite music can be healing. Also, showing photographs from different stages of the person's life can help to remind us that all lives change over time and that all lives end. Some memorial services invite the mourners to talk about the person, sometimes with advance notice and sometimes spontaneously.

It's a very good idea to honor the format that is chosen and to go along with whatever kind of service/memorial the person planning it has envisioned. For example, if only certain people have been asked to speak, it is not okay to add your voice to the formal part of the memorial service. There will likely be plenty of time afterward to share your memories informally with others who are grieving. On the other hand, if you are asked to speak at a memorial, it would be thoughtful to ask how long your tribute should be, how many others will be speaking, when in the service you will be asked to share your words in memory of the loved one, and to prepare your remarks in advance.

We have been to memorials where everyone was asked to wear Hawaiian shirts; where guests were encouraged to wear funny hats or running shoes to commemorate what the deceased valued. Whatever the planner thinks would have meaning and helps to recall happy moments from the deceased's life can be appropriate for a memorial service.

If food is included, and if the deceased was a vegan, having only vegan food at the memorial would be appropriate and honoring of the deceased. (When you write your will, you can request that only vegan food be offered at your memorial.)

Planning a funeral or a memorial service can keep us busy and distracted enough not to let the loss touch our most tender heart just yet. When the memorial or service is over, when the guests have left and you return to a new life in which a key element is missing, the hard work of grieving begins in earnest.

> If someone you loved dies, the love will survive the loss. "The passion of love bursting into flame is more powerful than death, stronger than the grave," says the Song of Solomon 8:6.

Mourning Is a Process

There is no time line for mourning and no predictable schedule. Even when we think we are finished grieving, a wave of grief can overpower us, seemingly out of the blue.

Although we may be given a day or a week off from work to mourn, mourning the loss of a loved one can take months, years, even a lifetime. One of the challenges of mourning is that others cannot tell that we are mourning. Often, if a few weeks have passed, our coworkers and friends presume that we are "back to normal," and that we ought to be "over it" already. Although we still want to talk about our loss, still want to share memories of the departed loved one, and describe the new seas that we now have to navigate without the loved one in our lives, others no longer want to listen. Their lives are moving forward while we may still feel mired in grief.

The twelve months after someone dies have been called "The Year of Firsts." Grief is intensified at the first birthday without your loved one; the first Thanksgiving; the first time anything you did together comes up and they are not with you. But these powerful bursts of renewed grief can happen years after your loss as well. Even when you think you are over your grief, waves of bereavement can return at any time, overwhelming you and knocking you off balance.

Beyond Mourning: Remembering Loved Ones

Relationships do not end when someone dies. For the rest of our lives we will continue to talk to this loved one, in our minds, on paper, or even aloud, and dream about them. Whenever Patti smells a cigar she says, "Hello, Daddy," as that unmistakable (and to her, repulsive) aroma reminds her of her father's loving presence in her life until she was in her forties. And when she makes potato pancakes at Hanukkah every year, she keeps a photo of her beloved grandmother nearby and speaks to her about how these potato pancakes are just like hers (minus the eggs). Her grandmother always made potato pancakes for Patti whenever she visited, and now they evoke loving memories of Grandma, keeping that relationship alive.

Over time, reminders of loved ones, such as photos and letters, can bring more comfort than tears (although the tears will still come at unexpected moments). Many people create small personal memorials to honor and remember people or animals

WHEN A CHILD DIES

When a child dies, at any age, parents experience a grief that is more devastating, and that lasts far longer, than for other types of losses. In the face of that unimaginable loss, it's difficult for friends and family to know what to do and say. It seems as though nothing could possibly ease the pain of this loss and most people feel helpless and inadequate.

The death of a child is a type of loss and mourning that is beyond the scope of this book. One helpful resource for grieving families and for those who wish to support those families is the Compassionate Friends website and publications. This nonprofit organization offers comfort, hope, and support for parents, siblings, and grandparents who have lost a child as well as guidance for those who wish to offer support and help. There are more than 660 chapters across the United States.

who have died. Patti's friend Peter was an avid gardener. He created a small shrine in the form of a circle of white rocks in his community garden plot. On each stone he wrote in black marker the name of a departed loved one. Every time he was tending the garden, the friends and family members he missed were there in his heart alongside him. Others who shared the community garden could also see this small shrine, and it invited conversation, giving Peter a chance to talk about people he had loved and lost.

Ginny's father used to tramp around in the snow in a pair of old-fashioned buckled galoshes. When he died, Ginny and her brothers took one of the galoshes up to the Maine woods where their family had vacationed for many years. They cut a hole in the bottom of a galosh and planted a tree. Although the galosh has mostly disintegrated and returned to the earth, every few years they take a trip to Maine to "visit Dad's boot."

Not all memories are wonderful, of course. If you and the deceased had a complicated relationship, if there were hard feelings left unresolved or unfinished business that causes you

A MOURNING PROCESS WITH ALL ITS
SLIDEBACKS AND SLOBTHROUGHS

Carol's artist friend Pamela, whose recommendations for caregivers we cite in chapter 4, described to Carol her mourning process after her husband died: "I tried to read myself through grief because I'd never done it before. I'd lost my parents, but it wasn't quite the same rawness of losing your partner."

The stages of death and dying actually refer to the dying person, not those who mourn after someone's death. Grief, Pamela says, "is so porous. It does get better in time in general, but then there are these slidebacks and slobthroughs." She found that there were about 20 to 30 "trigger songs" she has. "One or two notes of a song will send me right back."

Pamela attended a year of grief counseling offered through the hospice that supported them when her husband, Bill, was alive. She wrote her own "psalms," which were honest in the rawness of the grief expressed.

Because caregiving required her complete attention while Bill was alive, Pamela is rediscovering her friendships.

> The friends that I feel I can be real with, I spend more time with; those friendships have really deepened. I made some new friends, too. I laugh

with my friends quite a bit, but Bill and I would have laughed five times before we got up in the morning. I miss laughing because I am by myself. It's hard to break up at my own wit.

She recommends getting involved in volunteer work. This was another thing her caregiving had prevented her from doing. "With Bill so sick, he was my entire volunteer project." Her volunteer work is with children at two different Dallas schools and,

even if I am with them just twice a week, I think about them all the time. They are something to focus on in the here and now and not in the past. Volunteering, you get out of yourself. Instead of grief counseling that is trying to heal you, with volunteering you are helping others.

I had relinquished a lot of things because caregiving was so full time. I still have my artwork, but that's so solitary. But I have gotten out of the studio and I find that is real helpful. There are lots of different places that need us.

She suggested volunteering at an animal shelter would be meaningful as well.

Pamela and Bill were vegetarians. In the past year, she has become a vegan, and she feels this connects her to Bill, too. "I do feel he is very pleased that I have become a vegan again. He had no car, lived very simply, rode his bike, loved animals. He would be very happy that I'm living my life more ethically and compassionately."

distress, a bereavement-support group can be helpful for finding others who know what you are going through.

When an Animal Friend Dies
Animals living in the homes of vegans are, more often than not, ones who have been rescued. Not just from homelessness, but also from laboratories and even from food-production facilities. Although we vegans mourn the loss of our animal companions as much as anyone else, we experience a special type of comfort as well, knowing that the animal's life would have been so much less without us.

Ginny and her husband have cared for rescued cats, including older ones and those with special needs, for decades. Over the course of their 34 years of marriage, they have mourned the loss of 18 beloved cats. Friends will often ask, "How can you bear that much loss?" But for them, the loss is a necessary part of the joy that comes from sharing their lives with these animals. Although the grieving is always hard, there is comfort in knowing that each cat was saved from a difficult life as well as given a safe home and a loving, humane death.

Carol published a book called *Prayers for Animals* that offers comfort when an animal is suffering or dying, or even after they die. "Praying for animals allows us to unburden ourselves of these feelings by sharing them. In opening ourselves, we are kept open to the lives of others," she writes.

If a friend or family member loses a beloved animal, a gift in the animal's memory to any shelter or sanctuary would be a much-appreciated show of love. Sometimes others have no idea how closely bonded a human can be with a nonhuman animal friend. You may be the only person who understands the heartbreak of losing an animal friend. You may be the only person to whom they can express their deep sorrow.

And when your own animal companion dies, recognize that

you are grieving the loss of a beloved friend and treat yourself with the utmost tenderness. Ask friends to bear witness to your grief and to listen to you as you talk about your beloved animal. Be kind to yourself in the following weeks. You will never forget this special friend, and in the early days after your loss grief will greet you every time you come home, leave the house, and miss your buddy with a fully opened heart.

Some people keep photos of their deceased animal companions among family photos on display. Some people find that taking walks in the places the two of you used to walk can be soothing, albeit sad. Whatever it takes to mourn fully, find a way to do it. Mourning will help you reenter life when the time is right. Although you'll never be able to replace the being who is gone, after grieving for a while you may want to welcome another animal into your life for a new and different journey together.

When a Friend Is Mourning

As vegans, we are called to bring compassion to every being we encounter, and this is seldom more appropriate than when a friend of ours is mourning a loss. One of the best things we can do for a grieving friend is to listen. Let them talk about their loss, tell stories of the departed loved one, and be there to acknowledge their pain. We might also want to bring food, as people in grief often need to be reminded to eat. Nourishing vegan food is always appropriate, even if the friend is not a vegan.

Ask what organizations the deceased supported, and make a contribution in memory. Send a card to someone who is grieving. If you don't know what to say, there are countless commercial cards to express sympathy; though, on a blank card you could write, "I am holding you close in my heart" or "I am thinking of you and sending love." Even if your friend does not seem to respond to your card or call or food or visits, know that your kind words and actions are genuine gifts of love. Offering friendship and compassionate listening can be a lifeline for a friend in the depths of grief.

Another gift would be to check in regularly days, weeks, and months after a loss. Most people forget that grief continues, with new challenges, long after the memorial service. When others are tired of hearing about how this person is still mourning, your friendship and companionship can be invaluable.

How Animals Grieve

Recognizing that nonhuman animals grieve can help us feel more connected to the web of life and less isolated in our heartbreak.

More is known today than ever before about the emotional lives of animals. In 1995, Jeffrey Moussaieff Masson and Susan

While his white Sealyham terrier, Jennie, was dying, Maurice Sendak worked on the book *Higglety Pigglety Pop! Or, There Must Be More to Life.* He used a photograph of Jennie for illustration so that her shaggy jowls would be accurate. In the story, Jennie leaves her home, has a variety of experiences eating food and meeting animals, and becomes a nurse to a baby. She writes a letter to the human companion she left behind: "Hello, As you probably noticed, I went away forever. . . . I can't tell you how to get to Castle Yonder because I don't know where it is. But if you ever come this way, look for me. Jennie." Sendak's *In the Night Kitchen* includes a flour sack that reads "1953. Jennie. 1967 Bay Shore, L.I." Hints of Jennie can be found in the clock face with "Jennie" written on it. That book also includes references to his mother, and to his father, who was dying at the time Sendak was writing it. Sendak's amazing talent and creative genius allowed him to mourn, in part, through his work. ❧

McCarthy documented cases of horses, dogs, peregrine falcons, and other animals grieving when a partner died. They report these stories in the groundbreaking book *When Elephants Weep*, telling us, "The evidence of grief from other animal behaviors is strong."

We spoke with Jonathan Balcombe, director of animal sentience at the Humane Society of the United States and author of *What a Fish Knows*. He described how fish mourn the loss of a shoal mate or a tank mate.

> Fish can recognize individuals and can form life-long friendships with other fish. Farmed salmon show classic signs of depression, similar to what wild fish show when a favorite companion is suddenly gone. Often a fish will stop eating or swim vigil (circling the fish who died) for a few days after the loss of his companion.

When newborn calves are taken from their mothers on dairy farms, both the baby and the mother cry out for one another, look for one another frantically, and grieve for the broken bond they briefly experienced. When caged animals, like those at a zoo, are suddenly absent—whether by being transferred to another zoo or by dying—their cage mates exhibit grief. Monkey mothers have been seen carrying their dead children around.

Cynthia Moss describes how elephants may walk miles to return to a site where one of their family died. Elephant families return to touch the bones of a family member. When a matriarch named Big Tuskless died of natural causes, Moss described how she brought the elephant's jawbone to the research camp to determine her age at death:

> A few days after that, her family passed through the camp. There are several dozen elephant jaws on the ground in the

camp, but the family detoured right to hers. They spent some time with it. They all touched it. And then all moved on, except one. After the others left, one stayed a long time, stroking Big Tuskless's jaw with his trunk, fondling it, turning it. He was Butch, Big Tuskless's seven-year-old son.

More and more animal species have been discovered to form close bonds with other animals and to grieve the loss of these companions. Goats, buffalo, fish, elephants, birds, horses, chimpanzees, dogs, cats, and rabbits have all been known to mourn for those they have loved.

In her book *How Animals Grieve*, Barbara J. King gathers examples from cats to elephants to bunnies, goats, chimpanzees, and dolphins, and notes cross-species grieving as well. Like us, animals grieve because they have loved. "Grief does not respect species boundaries," writes King. She tells the story of Tarra, an elephant who became a close friend with a dog named Bella at the Elephant Sanctuary in Tennessee. When Bella was missing, apparently sick and dying, Tarra ate less and behaved in atypical ways. When Bella died, Tarra visited the gravesite for weeks.

Companion animals who share a home have been known to grieve the loss of a housemate of a different species as well.

If you live with a companion animal, you may know that when you return from an absence your dog is always delighted to see you, and your cat might "punish" you with distance at first. Both dogs and cats have been known to look for a deceased human caregiver for days or weeks or longer after they die. They also grieve for other animals in the household and may not have an appetite or want to play, and may look for the missing animal friend for quite a long time.

Animals share with us some of the same experiences when it comes to grief, suggesting that the disorientation, lack of appetite, and changed energy levels that come with acute grief are natural.

MOURNING AS A POLITICAL ACT

Philosopher and critical animal studies scholar James Stanescu, in writing about mourning as a political act, begins by situating us in a grocery store:

> In front of you is the violent reality of animal flesh on display: the bones, fat, muscles, and tissue of beings who were once alive but who have been slaughtered for the parts of their body. This scene overtakes you, and suddenly you tear up. Grief, sadness, and shock overwhelm you, perhaps only for a second. And for a moment you mourn, you mourn for all the nameless animals in front of you.

It is said that we all need public-mourning rituals, that "mourning requires other people." We live in the midst of a society that features the opposite of mourning rituals for animals: public rituals of celebration often center on dead animals (such as Thanksgiving and the Fourth of July). As vegans we experience a cruel, double disconnect: a society that celebrates what we grieve in a world that denies its actions and keeps grief itself at arm's length. Stanescu calls it "a strange, parallel world to that of other people" because,

> every day we are reminded of the fact that we care for the existence of beings whom other people manage to ignore, to unsee and unhear as if the only traces of the beings' lives are the parts of their bodies rendered into food: flesh transformed into

meat. To tear up, or to have trouble functioning, to feel that moment of utter suffocation of being in a hall of death is something rendered completely socially unintelligible. Most people's response is that we need therapy, or that we can't be sincere. So most of us work hard not to mourn. We refuse mourning in order to function, to get by. But that means most of us, even those of us who are absolutely committed to fighting for animals, regularly have to engage in disavowal.

In her essay "Facing Death and Practicing Grief," Lori Gruen explains how the fact that we mourn animals matters to our activism for animals. "The practices that lead to the suffering and death of other animals are practices that, in addition to causing pain and ending life, also render those lives meaningless. Developing counter-practices of mourning can help make those lives and, importantly, our relationships to those who are now gone, intelligible."

Mourning animals is truly a political act because it means that their lives mattered. Gruen suggests developing

a ritual vegan feasting practice, to share in our grief, to memorialize and mourn those who have died. The action at the National Animal Rights Day in which people silently hold dead animal bodies in a ritual of respect and mourning is an example of public mourning that refuses shame. ᕦ

We can remember that, as King says, there is no grief where there was no love. Regardless of what species is experiencing the loss of a friend, mourning and grief are the result of having loved. This fact can help us remember how fortunate we are to have known and loved another. It might help us remember that we are never alone in our grief.

All that Lives Must Die
We grieve because we love. Everyone who has experienced friendship, love, or closeness is susceptible to and capable of experiencing grief and mourning. As vegans, our circle of love and compassion is so huge that grieving is always with us. This empathy enables us to feel great compassion for others who are grieving. It's not an easy thing, this business of empathy and compassion. It can mean we end up shouldering a lot of the world's burden of sadness. That's why, when personal loss hits us, we need to turn our compassion toward ourselves. We need to choose for ourselves the time and resources that allow us to work through the process of grief and mourning.

Protecting Your Legacy of Kindness

WILLS, TRUSTS, AND OTHER LEGAL PROTECTIONS

EVERY ADULT NEEDS A WILL. WHETHER YOU CAN FIT ALL OF YOUR belongings into a shoebox or you have a house packed with fine antiques and a bank account to match, some things will need to be taken care of after you die. Your will specifies how you want those things addressed.

Without a will, those near to you have to guess what your wishes were. Or, if they knew your wishes, they might not be able to accomplish them without the legal authority a will provides. Vegan Anika Lehde, an activist in Seattle, shared a story about her uncle who died without a will.

> People who had been equally close to him had different opinions about what he wanted. Some cousins said he had promised to pay for their college education. There was confusion about what property should be left to whom, and there was disharmony and turmoil that has lasted for years. The family was thrown into disarray, and there was a lot of resentment when a single family member was deemed by law to be the sole heir.

Five years after his death, the family had still not healed. "There was permanent damage to the family," she reports.

Anika tells people that having a will is a gift of harmony for your family, and not having a will is one of the most selfish things a person can do. Anika created a will when she was in her twenties. She reasoned, "It's something adults do, and I'm an adult."

Having a will and making other legally binding arrangements can be especially meaningful for vegans. It's all a part of our legacy as animal advocates.

We'd like to think that our loved ones know us well enough to do right by us, but that isn't always the case. Imagine this: Aunt Edna knows you loved animals, so she makes a yearly donation to Heifer International (which gives animals used for food to people in the developing world) in your memory. How can you avoid this? By stating in your will and supporting documents where you want donations to go.

A will is absolutely crucial for ensuring that your companion animals will be cared for. It's also a place to specify what will happen to your vegan blog or other writings if that has been a part of your advocacy (your "intellectual property"). You want to make sure that veal medallions are not served at the lunch following your memorial service, right? And maybe you'd like to explore ways in which your remains can be treated so you aren't placing an undue burden on the environment and are, instead, protecting animal habitat.

Your impact on animals, your family and friends, and the world doesn't end when you die. But you won't be around to direct that impact. That's why you need a will.

In addition to a will, you'll need to create two documents that detail the kind of health care you desire if you become too sick to make health care choices for yourself. We discuss all of these documents below. Pulling them together is not difficult or expensive. An attorney can do it for you in just a few hours, and there are even cheaper ways to get this done.

The first step is to make several weighty decisions:

- What kind of health care do you want if you become too sick to make health care choices for yourself?
- Whom do you know who is trusted, capable, and can manage your personal and business affairs for you if necessary?
- Who will care for your animals while you are alive and also after you die?
- Who will serve as executor of your will?
- Where would you like memorial donations sent?
- What do you want done with your remains?

Once you've answered these questions, you're ready to get the legal documents you need to ensure your wishes are followed. Although you will probably create these documents at the same time, especially if you use an attorney, we will first address the documents that identify the kind of health care you wish while alive.

Health Care Decisions

We all hope for a quick, painless death in our sleep, but the vast majority of us don't end our lives that way. Part of your estate planning includes decisions about your medical care should you become incapacitated. Would you want your life prolonged if you are in a vegetative state? If you have a terminal illness, would you want extraordinary measures taken during a crisis? These discussions must occur in advance, and your choices must be put into writing and known to everyone who cares for you.

There are two types of documents you should have. The first is either an Advanced Health Care Directive (also called

Advanced Directive) or a POLST form. These documents provide guidance regarding your health care if you cannot speak on your own behalf. A POLST (Physician Orders for Life-Sustaining Treatment) form, also called a Living Will, addresses end-of-life care, specifically what kinds of heroic interventions are or are not wished. States may use different language to describe this form. When no heroic interventions are desired, this is called a DNR (Do Not Resuscitate). Whomever you name as your Durable Power of Attorney should have a copy of this document and so should your doctor. Bring a copy with you if you are taken to the hospital. Some people carry a card with this information in their wallet. This form ensures that your final hours or days will be spent as you choose.

The second document is a Durable Power of Attorney for Health Care (DPAHC) naming the person or persons who can make decisions for you. This document gives legal authority to another person to make health care decisions on your behalf. Ideally, this person would be making sure that your desire for heroic care (or not) is being followed. Should you be in an accident or have a condition that renders you unconscious or unable to communicate for any reason, you will need to have a trusted friend or family member in charge of following your wishes regarding your care. This person also will have the authority to release your body from a hospital to a mortuary.

Creating a Will

A will or a trust gives instructions and legal authority to your survivors and helps them take the next steps after you die. These legal documents allow you to decide who will inherit your property, whether that means a favorite necklace and electronic keyboard or a large house and everything in it. If you own anything at all that has value to you, no matter its financial value, or if you have children under the age of 18 or a partner to whom you are not legally married, you will want to have a will or a trust.

Dying without a will or a trust (dying "intestate" in legal terms) when you have any possessions, a partner to whom you are not married, or are responsible for the care of others (children, companion animals), has many negative results. Depending on the extent of your assets, the state will probably be able to claim more of them than they would if you'd had a will. Without a will, it may be hard for a partner to claim any property, even if it had only sentimental value.

If you do not have a will or trust, as noted, people may fight over who should inherit what and bicker over who will clean out your living space, who will close your bank accounts, and who will tell collectors to stop sending bills. Attorneys estimate that it will take years to resolve the estate left by Prince when he died without a will in 2016. Given how much he loved animals, think of the good his fortune might have done if he'd named a few animal rights organizations or sanctuaries in his will. You may not be a rich and famous rock star, but even a few hundred dollars makes a tremendous difference to an animal shelter, sanctuary, or educational nonprofit organization.

If you die without a will, somebody completely unknown to you or someone you would prefer not to delve into your business may end up going through your possessions, papers, medicine cabinet, drawers, and closets. This person will have to make multiple phone calls on your behalf: to a mortuary, to the cable company, to the utility company, to banks, and more. If this person is not aware in advance that this role will fall to them, they may even come to resent you, even as they mourn your passing, for leaving a mess for them to clean up in your absence.

To create a simple will you can hire an estate-planning attorney or do it yourself using a book or online resources. Chanel Reynolds, whose husband died before his will was signed, and who had to navigate his accounts and business in the midst of mourning, has become a champion of helping people create wills. Her excellent website, www.GYST.com (GYST stands for Get Your Shit Together), offers a review of many different companies that offer low-cost, online, legally valid will-creation services as well as Durable Power of Attorney for Health Care (DPOAHC).

If you do not want to do it yourself, you can hire an estate-planning attorney to help you prepare a will or trust, a DPOAHC, and an Advanced Health Care Directive. Don't be afraid to speak up about how much your beneficiaries (organizations and people to whom you are leaving assets) and animals mean to you. The attorney, whether or not an animal lover, will be sure that your instructions are clear and legally binding.

TYPES OF WILLS

A simple will is a written document that indicates how your property would be distributed when you die. You can revoke or change it at any time. It also allows you to appoint a guardian for any minor children.

In about half of the states in the U.S., wills can be as simple as a handwritten list of where you want your assets to go when you die. California requires that a handwritten will (also called a holographic will) be written entirely by you in your hand. You'll then have to have it notarized. There are additional legal requirements that vary by state, so be sure to consult a book about wills if you write one yourself. It is better to have this kind of will than not to have one at all. But it is better yet to use an online service, a book, or an attorney to create a more formal will that is valid in all fifty states.

Wills can be changed as often as you like. And given that none of us knows when we will die, it's best to create a will as soon as we can, regardless of what kind.

An alternative to a will is a *revocable living trust*. Usually prepared by an estate attorney, but also available from online companies and from books, a revocable living trust puts your property and assets "in trust" for someone else while you are alive. This means that the transfer of property after you die will go swiftly to your designated beneficiaries, often avoiding time in probate. It is similar to naming a beneficiary on a bank account. When you die, the named person is somewhat automatically the new owner of the account. (That person may still need to consult with an attorney.) An advantage of a living trust is that it can greatly reduce the time in probate and make the disposition of your assets happen more easily. If you have young children, the document also allows you to specify when you want them to inherit assets that are held in trust. A disadvantage is that a living trust must be actively managed. That means that any new assets you accrue have to be transferred into the trust. If you'd like to consider setting up a living trust, it's a good idea to talk first with an attorney to make sure it's the best choice for your needs.

Choosing an Executor

When you choose the person to be your executor, be sure to ask their permission first. This should entail a rather detailed conversation, as it's a significant responsibility. Choose someone you trust and someone who'll honor your wishes to the best of their ability.

The person you appoint (and an alternative, too, in case the first person cannot do this at the time of your death) should be named in your will. Again, this requires a conversation—or many, over time—to ensure that the responsibilities involved are understood completely.

In Case of Emergency

Always carry an ID with your name and the name and phone number of someone to call in case of emergency. A few years ago, a well-loved vegan runner was felled by an asthma attack that stopped his heart while he was running in cold weather. With no ID on him, he remained unidentified in a coma in a hospital for days before his family found him. When you are out and about, be prepared with information on your person— or on your smart phone if it's unlocked—so that another person can get you to a hospital, get your animals cared for, and take care of notifying your loved ones about what happened to you if you are in an accident. List your emergency contact as ICE (In Case of Emergency) in your smartphone address book. There are many ICE apps for smart phones. Most can be accessed even if your phone is locked.

If you have animals in your house, carry the name and number of someone who can get into your place and take the animals to care for them should you end up in a hospital. ✎

Passwords and Other Practical Concerns

When a friend of Patti's died recently, she was the executor of his estate. When she wanted to invite all his friends to the memorial, she went to his iPhone to look at his contacts list. Oops! The friend had his iPhone locked and nobody knew his password. Even the U.S. government cannot easily open an iPhone that is locked, and Patti certainly couldn't either. (The FBI paid $1 million to unlock the iPhone of the San Bernardino gunman. Patti did not do this with her friend.)

Estate planning attorney Kenneth Drexler helped us compile a checklist of the practical issues involved in preparing for your death. He stressed how critical it is that someone else knows where all of your essential information and documents can be found, including your will. This person may or may not be the executor of your will. Make sure that they are able to access your safe deposit box (although Kenneth recommends not keeping significant papers and information there, since it won't be immediately accessible, especially if the bank is closed) and that they also know where to find the following:

- Passwords for your phone, computer, and bank accounts
- Your date of birth and Social Security Number
- Your passport, birth certificate, title to your car and home; and where you keep your bank account/ retirement account/investment account and life-insurance information. Otherwise, someone will have to search and scramble through all your papers to find what they need when you're gone. (Know who was named on your bank accounts when you opened them as a contact person in case of your death; it may have been a long time ago when you opened the account, and this person may not still be the person you would choose today.)
- A list of your primary-care physician and other doctors with contact information for all
- Contact information for your family members
- Contact information for your bookkeeper, assistant, or tax preparer for your personal or business affairs, if you use these services
- Details about how you want to dispose of your body: this information can also be in your will, but it's good to make sure close friends or family members have access to the information as well.

Making Arrangements for Your Animals

If you have companion animals, assign someone now to be their guardian for when you are ill or dying and after you are gone. Do not presume that family members will take care of your animals as you would want them to. Perhaps they will, but the conversations must take place in advance of your illness and death. And if your animals are going to go to a home that already has animals living in it, you'll want to be sure that the new guardian can legally and safely keep your animals with the resident animals.

If you have the funds to do so, you may want to consider leaving some money for your animal caretaker. Know, however, that access to the funds in your estate may be blocked for a few weeks or months. Some states require as long as 90 days for legal proceedings before the executor is allowed to give away your money or possessions. Also, debts of your estate must be paid before beneficiaries receive whatever you left them. So think about giving some money to your future animal caretakers while you are alive and well. You might want to add their name to a small bank account so the funds can be used from day one for food, vet bills, and whatever other needs arise.

Be sure to provide specific instructions about your animals to their future caregiver. Write down and talk about any medical issues, the vet's name and contact information, health conditions, and anything else a caregiver should know. The more this person knows about your animal companions, the better they will be able to care for them.

Some auto insurance policies include protection for companion animals who may be hurt in a collision. Ask your insurance agent if this is available in your policy. Some veterinary costs, and sometimes even pet burial costs, may be included in the liability portion of your policy.

Protecting Your Intellectual Property

A respected vegan writer died without a will. As a result, the person who would have kept this author's books available had no ability to do so. If you are one of the many vegans maintaining blogs, writing zines, articles, and books, you may need to consider naming a *literary executor*.

This is someone who administers oversight of your literary production (published research, books, a blog, a website). They are responsible for maintaining copyright of your work, entering into contracts with publishers, collecting royalties for your heirs, and protecting your literary legacy.

Unless this person is your heir, they can act on your behalf only if given express authority to do so in your will. Perhaps your editor or agent has become a trusted friend. That person might make a good literary executor for you. Or maybe your family has an interest in your work and would look out for its integrity after you are gone. Then appoint someone to be your literary advocate and know that your work will be protected and/or promoted, as you would have liked.

Some libraries are actively collecting materials from the animal rights movement. If your papers, memorabilia, or collection of books and other printed material are to be archived after your death, you might want to consider starting that process while you are alive. Do you have a university that wants your work? Do you have a written agreement with them to accept it? Taking care of these details now will save your survivors a great deal of work and worry, protect your writings, and make available your collection for scholars and other activists.

Supporting Your Causes after You Die

Not only people but also organizations can be among the beneficiaries in your will or trust. If you want your savings to go to one or more favorite nonprofit organizations, you can name them as beneficiaries of your estate. You can designate either a specific amount or a percentage of your estate to be given to a charity or several charities, and this should be specified in your will or living trust. Many nonprofit organizations have legacy campaigns for this purpose. Although it's not necessary to let an organization know that you plan to leave them money, it helps them to know if you're going to continue your generosity when you're gone so they can sense whether they'll have funds in the future. By working with the legacy department or the attorney on staff at any organization(s) to which you plan to leave part of your estate, you can help ensure that your gifts will go where you want them to after you are gone.

You might also consider letting your executor know that you wish to ask for donations to a charity in lieu of flowers at your funeral or memorial service. Flowers for floral arrangements require energy for cultivation, transportation, and storage. Organic flowers still have large footprints and often are grown in soil that's been fertilized with animal blood or animal byproducts.

If for any reason you are not leaving anything to your family, you must make this explicit in your will. It is not enough simply to leave them out. Family members have sometimes gone to court to contest wills when they've been excluded. There are many ways to ensure that your assets go where you want them to if you are not leaving any to your family. One involves leaving them a small amount of money to show that you did remember them, but did not want to leave them more. Another involves language such as:

Except as otherwise provided in this Will, I have intentionally and specifically omitted to provide herein for any member of my family or their issue. After careful thought, disposition of my estate was made as herein set forth. If any court distributes any of my estate in a manner other than as directed herein, that court shall be acting in direct contradiction to my Will.

Other language indicates that someone contesting your will is to be excluded from it as a beneficiary:

If any person, whether a beneficiary or not, in any manner, directly or indirectly, contests or attacks this Will, or any of its provisions, any share or interest in my estate given to the contesting person under this Will is revoked and shall be disposed of in the same manner as if that contesting person had predeceased me without issue.

Even an ironclad will can be contested. This rarely happens, but it is certainly worth knowing about. A fascinating 2009 documentary film called *The Art of the Steal* is about an art collector whose will stipulated clearly what he wanted for his collection of valuable paintings after he died. Despite many well-respected, highly paid attorneys, his wishes were not honored in the end. So it might be wise to consider giving away as much as you can before you die, while you are still in control of your gifts. The less that is left to distribute when you're gone, the fewer opportunities for contested wills, fighting over inheritances, and ill-will among your survivors.

An added bonus of giving your gifts when you are alive is that your generosity can help simplify your life. Downsizing and simplifying are gratifying in and of themselves. The joy of supporting causes you love, added to the joy of living simply, are gifts you can give to yourself when you are alive and well. Also, we can enjoy the benefits of our generosity more fully by giving when we are alive. It may be helpful to meet with a financial adviser to determine how much you can safely donate while ensuring that your own future needs are covered.

There are very few things we can do on Earth after we die. But sharing our wealth with good organizations is one way to prolong our legacy of caring even beyond our life.

⊰ 8 ⊱

Last Words, Organ Donations, and Resting Places

H OW WOULD YOU LIKE TO BE REMEMBERED WHEN YOU'RE GONE?
Wouldn't you like to have a say in shaping your legacy?
One way to do so is to write your own obituary or leave notes
for whoever will be responsible for writing it. Even if you
don't expect to die any time soon, it's an interesting exercise
in clarifying your values, remembering the high and low
points in your life, and suggesting to your survivors how
you'd like to be thought of when you are gone. As Barbara J.
King writes in *How Animals Grieve*,

> Like a hall of mirrors, an obituary illuminates in our
> imagination not only the person now lost, but also a
> life that echoes (and echoes again) across time and
> space. In it we read the names of those who died before
> and the survivors, the past and future in unbroken
> continuity.

If you're a regular reader of obituaries, you know that
a well-written one can read like an interesting story. It is
fascinating to see how eight or more decades of life can be
summarized in a few paragraphs. And it's a lesson in the
unpredictable nature of death to see how many people die

"before their time." That phrase is interesting, because life offers no guarantees regarding longevity.

We can find inspiration in obituaries by reading about the challenges others faced. We can develop empathy and wake up to the truth of our own mortality by getting into the habit of reading the obits in any paper. We can also be reminded about what means most in our lives and recognize aspects of our lives worth remembering.

Think about how you'd like to be remembered. Are there accomplishments you are proud of? Are there people or animals who meant the world to you? People or events that helped to shape you or guide you in your life? Were there challenges you met with courage? Or with fear, but overcame them anyway? Write a list of favorite memories and fervent wishes, regrets, and dreams, whether realized or not. Suggesting what you might want mentioned in your obituary will be a tremendous help to those who survive you. This list can also identify the organizations to which you'd like people to make gifts in your memory. And it can remind your survivors that you want only vegan food served at any memorial service or on your birthday every year, or any time they want to remember and honor your life.

WRITING A LIFE REVIEW LETTER

Writing a letter to loved ones is another option for sharing your thoughts and feelings about your life with family and friends. The Stanford Palliative Care Education and Training Program has developed a template to help you write a letter for those you will one day leave behind. Whereas some people write this letter when they are already nearing death, many choose to write it when they are well, sometimes updating it as needed, year by year.

The letter guides you in completing seven tasks of life review:

Task 1: Acknowledge the important people in your life.

Task 2: Remember treasured moments from your life.

Task 3: Apologize to those you love if you hurt them.

Task 4: Forgive those who love you if they have hurt you.

Task 5: Express your gratitude for all the love and care you have received.

Task 6: Tell your friends and family how much you love them.

Task 7: Take a moment to say "good-bye."

For more information about how to complete these tasks, visit the Stanford Friends and Family Letter Project online. ⌐

Becoming an Organ Donor

When you become an organ donor, you have the potential to save up to eight lives, and through donation of skin tissue, corneas, and other parts of the body, to improve the lives of many other people. For some vegans, though, this raises ethical concerns. If your organs go to saving the lives of meat eaters, aren't you contributing to the deaths of more animals?

Although this might be true, a vegan ethic is really more complicated than this. As vegans, we want to contribute to a more compassionate and just world. But we do this by changing hearts and habits, not by wishing for harm to meat eaters. Most of us include non-vegans within our circle of loved ones. We cherish their lives and wouldn't want any of them to die for lack of a donated organ. Being an organ donor is part of an ethic of generosity and compassion; it's a very vegan decision.

In fact, it's even possible to donate certain organs while you're still alive and in that case, you may even get to determine who gets the organ. Animal activist Hillary Rettig donated one of her kidneys to a complete stranger. She was able to choose her recipient through a database of people with kidney disease. She chose a retired veterinarian who runs a no-kill animal shelter.

Organ donation is one way to let your body keep working for others after you are gone. Another option is to donate your body to scientific research.

Willing Your Body to Science
Although willing your body to science has been the least-common choice for dealing with remains, it's becoming more popular. Georgetown University, the University of Minnesota, Duke University, the University of Arizona, and the University of Buffalo all reported an increase of bodies donated in recent years according to a 2016 Associated Press story. The operations director at the Georgetown University body-donation program reported that the combination of saving money and the lifting of old taboos accounted for the surge in donations. "It's just a priceless donation," according to a professor of surgery at Duke University.

At University of California at San Francisco, after the body is used for classes, it may be cremated and the cremains are scattered at sea. Some universities return the body to the family after it has been used in classes. Despite the environmental impact of cremation, donating your body for medical science may end up saving the lives of other animals, and will certainly contribute to the education of future doctors.

Choices about Your Remains

Visiting a mortuary, choosing a cemetery or crematorium, and making plans for your own death are surprisingly satisfying endeavors. Making these arrangements in advance will ease the burden on the people you love when they are grieving your death. It is a beautiful gift to give to your survivors. At a time when they are least prepared to make business decisions, they will be free to mourn your loss and celebrate your life without having to choose a casket, arrange a cremation, or buy a burial plot, and fret over whether or not you would have liked their choices. It's also another way to exercise some control now, given that we don't know if we'll have any say at all as we approach our death.

In the United States today, burial and cremation are the only two common legal ways to dispose of bodies after death. Neither method is ideal for the health of the planet.

Although by far the more popular choice today, cremation requires 45–90 minutes of temperatures between 1,300 and 1,800 degrees Fahrenheit to reduce a human body to ash and mineral fragments. The fire burns natural gas, releasing greenhouse gases. Additionally, cremation releases chemicals such as dioxins and furans into the atmosphere. When people have mercury fillings in their teeth, vaporized mercury is released as well. Even when cremation is chosen, some sort of combustible container is usually necessary to hold the body. We can reduce the impact of cremation by choosing caskets made from unpainted wood, wicker, or recycled cardboard and by being cremated in a shroud of linen or cotton rather than synthetic clothing. If someone is going to bury the ashes, we can choose a biodegradable urn.

Conventional burials also hurt our land. Embalming, polished caskets, steel vaults, tombstones, and cut flowers that are part of modern burials in developed countries take a toll on the environment. Lacquered woods and metal caskets leave a huge carbon footprint. And 800,000 gallons of formaldehyde-based embalming fluids are buried in U.S. cemeteries every year. Although state laws vary on this, most allow you to forego embalming unless there are certain highly contagious diseases involved.

Green Burials
A green burial uses a coffin made from biodegradable wood, wicker, or cardboard without paint or lacquer. Or you may be buried in only a shroud, sometimes fitted with wood panels or handles. There is no embalming and no tombstone. According to the Green Burial Council, green burials reduce carbon emissions, protect workers' health, conserve natural resources, and preserve habitat. For more information about green burials and to find a cemetery that has green burials, go to greenburialcouncil.org.

There are a number of additional, innovative options for green burials on the horizon. Designers in Italy have proposed a biodegradable, egg-shaped pod to take the place of an urn for ashes or a casket for bodies. Called Capsula Mundi, the pod is used to fertilize a tree that is to be planted above it and that serves as a living memorial to the deceased instead of a stone headstone. The trees in this new kind of cemetery are referred to as a sacred forest.

Another creative option is a burial suit, which is already available. Made from a unique strain of mushrooms, the suit itself can improve the health of soil. See the Sources and Further Reading section at the end of this book for more information about these options for green burials.

Whole-Family Cemeteries and Green Pet Burials
Traditional options for a simple burial of a pet include a pet cemetery or a DIY burial in your yard. But cultural

anthropologist Eric Greene, who founded the Green Pet-Burial Society (GreenPetBurial.org), says the concept of a pet cemetery is misleading. "While cemeteries designed for human remains are usually protected in perpetuity, most pet 'cemeteries' are not so protected despite the assurances given by some pet cemetery owners."

For this reason, many pet cemeteries insist upon using plastic or metal caskets for easier disinterment, preventing the body from reintegrating with the natural environment.

There are many problems with DIY burials at home or in parks and wilderness areas as well, according to Greene. These include legal and zoning issues (and the possibility of future development); digging a deep-enough grave (so that animals don't dig up the remains); and the effect on future owners of a home. "The new owners might excavate the land for new landscaping, a pool, an extension or new building—or it may eventually be 'developed' for some other use," says Greene.

Regarding burial in public parks, there is always a possibility that rangers may catch you, or may come across a freshly dug grave and want to investigate. The question is—why should anyone in their bereavement need to sneak around or take risks in order to give their beloved a proper burial?

The Green Pet Burial Society is working to normalize conservation through whole-family cemeteries. In a whole-family cemetery, remains of pets may be interred alongside human family members within a wildlife habitat. The tagline for this program is "together in death as in life." Right now, whole-family cemeteries can be found in just a handful of states; the Green Pet Burial Society continues to advocate for legislation to expand choices.

Burying animals and humans together is nothing new. Anthropologist Robert Lose, who studies human–dog relationships, states, "As soon as we see skeletal remains that look like the modern dog—say 14,000 years ago—we see dogs being buried [alongside human remains]." Greene says, "By promoting conservation whole-family cemeteries we are helping to broaden the concept of 'family' and raise the status of all animals."

⊰ Afterword ⊱

A Vegan Understanding of Death

ALLAN KELLEHEAR'S *A SOCIAL HISTORY OF DYING* PROVIDES AN overview of how cultures have viewed dying over the millennia. He finds that in contemporary culture there is an *erosion of awareness of dying* as well as an *erosion of support for dying*. In addition, there is a problem of stigma attached to dying. Besides the stigma, the topic and reality of death provoke much anxiety. We see it in people's responses to those who are gravely ill and dying. Whereas most people don't want to think about their deaths, for us vegans there really is something more at stake. Our veganism is about combatting anti-animal attitudes in our culture. Could our reluctance to acknowledge our future deaths be linked to that? According to some philosophers, our denial of death might relate directly to the status of animals in our culture.

Some scholars have suggested that our fear of death is one reason we separate ourselves from nature and animals. In their article "Denial of Death and the Relationship between Humans and Other Animals," Lori Marino and Michael Mountain write, "When we humans are reminded of our personal mortality, we tend to deny our biological identity or creatureliness and distance ourselves from the other animals, since they remind us of our own mortal nature."

We express this distance in so many ways and even in the language used to describe the attributes we share in common with animals. We cultivate friendships, *they* have "affiliative behavior"; we love, *they* mate; we use our intelligence, *they* are instinctive. This belief that we are different from (and better than) other animals is known as human exceptionalism.

Human exceptionalism creates the justification for treating the other animals however we, the humans, wish. Marino and Mountain argue that, "killing and wielding power over animals gives us power over the life and death of another, creating the illusion of our own immortality." Meat eaters, for instance, have the power over the life and death of animals by choosing to eat them.

Vegans actively challenge this power over the other animals by choosing not to eat them. And our activism may be enhanced when we recognize that this power, and the resistance to giving it up, is, in part, tied to fear of death.

Dr. Robert Pogue Harrison of Stanford University also discusses a connection between the denial of death and the killing and eating of animals, dairy, and eggs. In his book *The Dominion of the Dead*, he argues that individuals belonging to the current generation are the first to have no idea where they will be buried when they die. He also claims that this generation is unique in not knowing where our food comes from. We're in denial about both our death and about how animal food is produced, and Harrison believes these are related. He writes that, until recently,

> the great majority of human beings lived and toiled on the land where their ancestors were interred, where they and their children and their children's children would also be interred. This is no longer the case in Western societies. For the first time in millennia, most of us don't know where we will be buried, assuming we will be buried at all.

He adds:

It goes hand in hand with another indeterminacy that until recently would have been equally unthinkable for the majority. Most of us have no idea where the food we eat comes from. We are oblivious of the fields that yielded our grain, the gardens our vegetables sprouted in, the orchards where our fruits are gathered. We are not familiar with the individual animals we eat: we don't tend to them, we don't watch them grow, we don't know what flock they came from or on which pastures they grazed, and above all we have no hand in their sacrifice. The daily holocausts that supply the world markets' demands for meat, fish, and poultry take place in another world than the one most of us inhabit. And yet we live off such holocausts, inevitably.

In *The Sexual Politics of Meat,* Carol identifies the structure of the *absent referent* to explain how animals disappear literally and metaphorically in meat eating. Behind every meal of meat is an absence: the death of the nonhuman animal whose place the meat takes. When people eat meat, the absent referent separates the consumer from the consumed, from the animal who died. Humans do not regard meat eating as contact with another animal; it is simply seen as contact with food. Who is suffering? No one, it seems.

Harrison suggests that the absent referent allows us not only to remain unaware of where our food comes from, but also to remain in denial about our own death. He says:

> When the "from" of the things we consume becomes not only remote but essentially unreal, the world we live in draws a veil over the earth we live on—a veil that obscures not only the source of our foodstuffs but also the source of our relation to the earth, namely our death.

Awareness of our dying confronts us with the limits of our bodies. Eating as healthfully as possible and striving to manage our weight—to achieve some sort of "vegan ideal" body (that is, in fact, culturally determined and loaded with sexist and ableist presumptions) is a way of controlling something that is really not within our control. We might exercise and diet down to a certain weight (or at least some of us can) and eat in a way that reduces risk for disease, but eventually we have no control over the death of our body. In believing that we do, we've made of our own death an absent referent, allowing ourselves to ignore it. We foster the view that we hold dominion over death, and consequently over those who remind us of it: the animals.

We Are Animals Who Will Die
If our human exceptionalism is related to, as James Stanescu says, "a fear and shame that we are, in fact, nothing but animals," what is the remedy?

To begin with, we can normalize death by taking our future deaths seriously enough to create the necessary legal documents that death and dying require. We also normalize death by finding ways to be comfortable with and support those who are dying. But that's just a start.

Human exceptionalism is reinforced by meat, dairy, and egg consumption. Vegans challenge our culture's denial of animals' death. Why, therefore, have vegans not been in the forefront of challenging the general denial of death that undergirds a denial of our animality? We may simply be mirroring and enacting our culture's position. We, too, end up repressing the knowledge of death as a way to hold our anxiety about death at bay. If we saw acceptance of our death and its corollary—the needed preparation for this eventuality—as part of our vegan activism and living, would we find it easier to accept our future deaths and act accordingly? Perhaps the next step for vegan activism is to model a different way, not just in relationship to animals, but to death.

⊰ Acknowledgments ⊱

Thank you first and foremost to you, the reader, for staying with us throughout this book, one that raises difficult issues that most of us would rather not look at.

Thank you to Martin Rowe, our editor and publisher, who believed in our message from the start and embraced it fully. At a pivotal moment, Andy Ross offered guidance and we thank him for his time and wisdom. Dr. Michael Greger gave generously of his time in providing our book's foreword. We're grateful for his contribution and for all of his work aimed at keeping vegans healthy. Thank you to attorney Kenneth Drexler for his expert guidance on estate planning. We thank Barbara King and Jonathan Balcombe for taking the time to talk with us about how animals grieve and for their important work and books about animal sentience and emotions. And thank you to Eric Greene who generously shared information about green pet burials.

Thank you to Jo Anna, Lisa, Janet, Lisa, Scott, Caela, Rachael, and Ellen for being willing to share thoughts and experiences that were fundamental in helping us shape our message. We also gleaned insight and wisdom from vegan bloggers, especially Laura Wright, Eric Polsinelli, Anika Lehde, Susan Voisin, and Paul Shapiro.

We're grateful for the valuable views on caregiving that Carol's friend Pamela Nelson shared so generously. We thank two incredible vegan caregivers, Donna Rhodes and Donna

Marino, for reflecting on their caregiving experiences and offering insights and suggestions based on their loving care of a vegan activist.

From Carol
Thank you to Lori Gruen, Sunny Taylor, Josephine Donovan, and James Stanescu for their invaluable work in the field of critical animal studies, the ethics of care, caregiving, and mourning. And to Pamela Nelson not only for sharing her experiences as a caregiver and then as someone grieving, but for all the death and dying books she passed on to me. For his patience as I tackled yet another book project and for his understanding as we got out our wills to update them, thanks to Bruce A. Buchanan.

From Patti
Thank you to Fran Zitner and Stan Rosenfeld, for their ongoing, unconditional support; Anna Douglas for her beautiful teachings on the Buddhist understanding of aging, illness, and dying; estate-planning attorneys, whose work is noble; and all my friends and family members who have prepared their wills.

From Ginny
Thank you to my blog readers who generously provided stories, insights, and experiences about what it is like to live as a vegan with a chronic disease. I'm also strengthened and inspired by the growing community of vegan dietitians whose own messages about animals and about nutrition and health align with the messages of this book. Thank you especially to Jack Norris, RD; Reed Mangels, PhD, RD; Matt Ruscigno, MPH, RD; Anya Todd, RD; Carolyn Tampe, MS, RD; Taylor Wolfram, MS, RD; David Weinman, RD; and Ed Coffin, RD. Finally, and as always, I am blessed to be married to Mark Messina, best nutrition adviser, best cat dad, and best husband.

⊰ Sources and Further Reading ⊱

1. When Vegans Get Sick
Plant-based Diets and Health
- EPIC–Oxford Study: epic-oxford.org/
- The Adventist Health Study-2: publichealth.llu.edu/adventist-health-studies
- The American Institute for Cancer Research: wcrf.org/int/research-we-fund/our-cancer-prevention-recommendations

Body Shaming and Stigma
- Amy Farrell, *Fat Shame: Stigma and the Fat Body in American Culture.* New York: New York University Press, 2011.
- Laura Wright: veganbodyproject.blogspot.com/2016/09/hillarys-health-and-my-heart-attack.html

Vegan Nutrition
- Veganhealth.org
- TheVeganRD.com/vegan-nutrition-primers
- Vegetariannutrition.net

2. How Shame and Blame Affect Our Health and Our Advocacy
Vegans and Chronic Disease
- Susan Voisin: blog.fatfreevegan.com/2014/10/my-unexpected-diagnosis.html
- Sarah Kramer: blog.govegan.net/bad-news/
- Eric Posinelli: https://www.veganostomy.ca/about-me/

OTHER REFERENCES
- Canadian Obesity Network: obesitynetwork.ca/public

3. A Vegan Ethic of Care

Developing a vegan ethic of care draws on the important work of feminists in articulating a feminist ethic of care, specifically *The Feminist Care Tradition in Animal Ethics*, an anthology edited by Carol and Josephine Donovan, published by Columbia University Press.

OTHER REFERENCES
- Debra Roppolo, "The Crime of Indifference," theseglasswalls. wordpress.com/2016/10/05/the-crime-of-indifference/
- The quotations from Sunaura Taylor and Eva Kittay are from Taylor's "Interdependent Animals: A Feminist Disability Ethic-of-Care," in Carol J. Adams and Lori Gruen, *Ecofeminism: Feminist Intersections with Other Animals and the Earth.* New York: Bloomsbury, 2014. Taylor's *Beasts of Burden: Animal and Disability Liberation* was published by The New Press in 2017.
- Lori Gruen, *Entangled Empathy.* New York: Lantern, 2015.
- Simone Weil, *Waiting on God.* London: Fontana, 1951/1971.
- Heather Plett, "What It Really Means to Hold Space for Someone": http://upliftconnect.com/hold-space/ (May 8, 2016)

4. When Someone You Love Is Seriously Ill or Dying

- Susan Sontag, *Illness as Metaphor.* New York: Farrar, Straus & Giroux, 1971.
- Tom Lubbock, *Until Further Notice, I Am Alive.* London: Granta, 2014.
- Steven Thrasher, "Don't Tell Cancer Patients What They Could Be Doing to Cure Themselves," *Guardian*, March 26, 2016: theguardian.com/commentisfree/2016/mar/26/do-not-tell-cancer-patients-cures-they-could-be-doing
- Susan Silk and Barry Goldman, "How Not to Say the Wrong Thing," *Los Angeles Times*, April 7, 2013: articles.latimes.com/2013/apr/07/opinion/la-oe-0407-silk-ring-theory-20130407

- The section on "different laws" for caregiving is taken from Carol's article "Toward a Philosophy of Care through Caregiving," *Critical Inquiry*, Summer 2017.
- Pamela Nelson's TEDxSMU talk: tedxtalks.ted.com/video/When-caregiving-comes-your-way;TEDxSMU
- Marion Couts, *The Iceberg*. New York: Grove, 2016.

5. When You Have a Terminal Illness

- Katherine Russell Rich, *The Red Devil: To Hell with Cancer—and Back*. New York: Crown, 1999.
- Paul Shapiro, "Lisa Shapiro: 1964–2015. Advocating for Animals Right up to Her Final Moments": cok.net/lisa-shapiro/
- Caring Bridge: visit caringbridge.org/
- *Five Wishes*: thelastvisit.com/resources/advance-directives/five-wishes-a-planning-tool/ and from Aging with Dignity: agingwithdignity.org/five-wishes/five-wishes-online
- Sherwin Nuland, *How We Die: Reflections of Life's Final Chapter*. New York: Vintage, 1995.
- For helping to plan for the end of life: blog.sevenponds.com/

6. Mourning

- Barbara J. King, *How Animals Grieve*. Chicago: University of Chicago Press, 2013.
- Patricia Kelley, *Companion to Grief: Finding Consolation When Someone You Love Has Died*. New York: Simon & Schuster, 1997.
- C. S. Lewis, *A Grief Observed.* New York: HarperOne, 2001.
- Kelli Swazey, TED talk: ted.com/talks/kelli_swazey_life_that_doesn_t_end_with_death?language=en
- For families who have lost a child: CompassionateFriends.org
- Carol J. Adams, *Prayers for Animals.* New York: Continuum, 2004.
- Information on Maurice Sendak from Katie Roiphe, *The Violet Hour.* New York: Dial, 2016.
- Jeffrey Moussaieff Masson and Susan McCarthy, *When Elephants Weep.* New York. Delacorte, 1995.
- Jonathan Balcombe, *What a Fish Knows.* New York: Farrar, Straus & Giroux, 2016.

- Cynthia Moss, *Elephant Memories: Thirteen Years in the Life of an Elephant Family*. Chicago: University of Chicago Press, 2000.
- James Stanescu, "Species Trouble: Judith Butler, Mourning, and the Precarious Lives of Animals." *Hypatia* 27: no. 3 (August 2012): 567–82.
- Lori Gruen, "Facing Death and Practicing Grief," in *Ecofeminism: Feminist Intersections with Other Animals and the Earth*, ed. Carol J. Adams and Lori Gruen. New York: Bloomsbury. 2014.
- Pauline Laurant lost her husband in the Vietnam War when she was pregnant with their first child. Because of the unpopularity of that war, she was ashamed to tell people how her husband died. So she did not properly mourn her loss for decades. Instead, she moved from one addiction to another trying to dull the ache that pervaded her. Years later, she learned to accept fully the magnitude of her loss, allowing her grief to surface and be acknowledged, and healed through grieving. Her story about the importance of grieving is told in her memoir, *Grief Denied*: griefdenied.com/summary.html

7. Protecting Your Legacy of Kindness
ESTATE PLANNING AND ADVANCE DIRECTIVES

- Caring Info: caringinfo.org
- National POLST Paradigm: polst.org/
- Get Your Shit Together: GYST.com

8. Last Words, Organ Donations, and Resting Places

- Stanford Friends and Family Letter Project: med.stanford.edu/letter/about.html
- To learn more about green burials: greenburialcouncil.org
- To learn more about the environmental impact of a standard American funeral: sevenponds.com/after-death/environmental-impact-of-death
- For directories on green cemeteries and conservation whole-family cemeteries: GreenPetBurial.org
- See "Researcher Explores Close Relationship between Human and Dog": heritagedaily.com/2016/03/researcher-

explores-close-prehistoric-relationship-between-human-and-dog/109905
- Hillary Rettig wrote about her donation on the *Huffington Post*: http://www.huffingtonpost.com/hillary-rettig/my-big-fat-vegan-kidney-d_b_163139.html

Afterword

- Allan Kellehear, *A Social History of Dying*. Cambridge: Cambridge University Press, 2007.
- Lori Marino and Michael Mountain, "Denial of Death and the Relationship between Humans and Other Animals," *Anthrozoös: A Multidisciplinary Journal of the Interactions of People and Animals*. 28: no. 1 (April 2015): 5–21.
- Robert Pogue Harrison, *The Dominion of the Dead*. Chicago: University of Chicago Press, 2003.
- Carol J. Adams, *The Sexual Politics of Meat: A Feminist-Vegetarian Critical Theory*. New York: Bloomsbury. 1990/2015.

⊰ Index ⊱

Fat Shame (Farrell), 9
fat stigma. *See* body shaming
fecal immunochemical test (FIT), 20
feminism, 38
fish, 85
Five Wishes, 57, 66–67
food: care teams and, 55, 56; denial of death and, 113–14; grief and, 83; in hospitals, 55, 56, 65; at memorial services, 77, 105. *See also* diet and health
funerals/memorials, 74–80; burial/cremation, 107–11; flowers at, 101; memory and, 78–80; participation in, 76–77; religious, 74–76. *See also* death

gender: body shaming and, 9; compassion and, 35–36; heart disease and, 5, 11–12; MS and, 17; sexism, 15, 38, 115
genetics, 6, 11, 14, 15, 29
Georgetown University, 107
Goldman, Barry, 49–50
Green Burial Council, 109
Greene, Eric, 110
Green Pet-Burial Society, 110
grief. *See* mourning/grief
Gruen, Lori, 37–38, 88
guaiac-based fecal occult blood test (gFOBT), 20
Guardian, 46

Hall, Martha Murphy, 75
Harrison, Robert Pogue, 113–14
health care, 91–93. *See also* diet and health; hospitals
heart disease, 5, 10–12, 13
HIPAA (Health Insurance Portability and Accountability Act), 52

holding space, 38–39, 40
hospice, 65
hospitals: emergency contacts and, 97; food at, 55, 56; health care documents, 91–93; pets in, 65. *See also* medicine
How Animals Grieve (King), 72, 86, 104
How We Die (Nuland), 71
Huffington Post, 28
Humane Society of the United States, 85
human exceptionalism, 113, 115
hypertension, 5

Iceberg, The (Couts), 55
identity, 31–32
ill, caring for the, 42–58; care teams, 51–58; etiquette, 42–48; hospice and, 65; living wills and, 66–67
illness, 61–71; autonomy and, 41; communication about, 64–65; coping with, 62–64; guilt/shame about, 68–70; identity and, 31–32; shaming of, 24–26, 68. *See also* cancer; care; diet and health; ill, caring for the; mourning
Illness as Metaphor (Sontag), 42
Independent, 45
inflammation, 13, 16, 17, 18
insulin, 16
insurance, 99
intellectual property, 100
interdependency, 36–38, 41
Islam, 76

Jobs, Steve, 25–26
Joisher, Kuntal, 68
Judaism, 76

Kellehear, Allan, 112
Kelley, Patricia, 73–74

rituals. *See* funerals/memorials
Roppolo, Debra, 35

saturated fat, 16, 17
Sendak, Maurice, 84
sexism, 15, 38, 115
Sexual Politics of Meat (Adams),
    114
shame/blame, 21–22, 24–32;
    care shaming, 35–36, 37, 38;
    depression and, 13, 14; for
    diseases, 24–26, 42–43; grief
    and, 88; self-blame, 27–28;
    unsolicited advice and,
    26–27; vegan community,
    effectiveness of, and, 30–32.
    See also body shaming
Shapiro, Lisa, 56, 62–63, 64
Shapiro, Paul, 62–63
sigmoidoscopy, 20
Silk, Susan, 49–50
skin, 14–15, 21
sleep, 18
smoking, 10
Social History of Dying (Kellehear),
    112
social life, 6
social media, 44, 47, 56, 63
Sontag, Susan, 42
soy, 14
Stanescu, James, 87–88, 115
Stanford Palliative Care
    Education and Training
    Program, 105–6
Stool DNA test (sDNA), 20
stress, 6, 10, 18, 26, 29–30
Strydom, Maria, 68
Swank Diet, 17
Swazey, Kelli, 74

Taylor, Sunaura, 36–37
therapy, 14
Thrasher, Steven, 46–47
Todd, Anya, 22

trans fat, 16
trust, living, 96

University of California at San
    Francisco, 107

veganism: as panacea, 21–23, 24–
    25; values/ethic of, 30, 70–71,
    106–7. *See also* activism;
    shame/blame
Vegan Society, 69
vegetarians, 5, 11–12, 13
vitamin D, 17
Voisin, Susan, 25, 27

weight: body shaming, 8–9,
    18, 29–30, 30–32; diabetes
    and, 12; diet and, 5, 29, 115;
    obesity, 8–9. *See also* body
    shaming
Weil, Simone, 38
What a Fish Knows (Balcombe), 85
When Elephants Weep (McCarthy,
    Masson), 85
wills, 66–67, 77, 90–103; animals
    and, 91, 99; charities and,
    101–3; contesting of, 101–2;
    creation of, 94–95; executor
    of, 96, 99, 100; importance
    of, 90–92, 93–94; intellectual
    property and, 100; types of,
    95–96
World Cancer Research Fund, 7
Wright, Laura, 11

⊰ About the Authors ⊱

Carol J. Adams, MDiv, is the author of the pioneering *The Sexual Politics of Meat*, called a "vegan bible" by the *New York Times* (now in a twenty-fifth anniversary Bloomsbury Revelations edition), plus many other books. *The Carol J. Adams Reader* appeared in 2016. She frequently speaks on college campuses. She is working on a memoir about her decade as a caregiver. She lives near Dallas, Texas, with her partner and their two rescued dog companions, Holly and Inky. Find out more about Carol at caroljadams.com.

Patti Breitman is the director of the Marin Vegetarian Education Group, and a cofounder of Dharma Voices for Animals. She is the coauthor with Connie Hatch of *How to Say No without Feeling Guilty*, and with Carol J. Adams of *How to Eat like a Vegetarian Even if You Never Want to Be One*. Patti is on the advisory councils of the Animals & Society Institute and Jewish Veg. In 2016 she was awarded the Lisa Shapiro Award for Unsung Vegan Heroes. Patti and her husband advocate for people and animals in need of support in the San Francisco Bay Area.

Virginia Messina, MPH, RD, is coauthor of *Vegan for Life* and *Vegan for Her*, and of the first textbook on vegetarian nutrition for medical professionals. She writes and speaks on vegan nutrition for both consumers and health professionals. Ginny serves on the board of directors of Vegfund and on advisory boards of One Step for Animals, Veg Youth, and the Vegetarian Resource Group. She lives in Pittsfield, Massachusetts, with her husband and an ever-changing population of rescued cats. Find out more about Ginny at TheVeganRD.com.

⊰ About the Publisher ⊱

LANTERN BOOKS was founded in 1999 on the principle of living with a greater depth and commitment to the preservation of the natural world. In addition to publishing books on animal advocacy, vegetarianism, religion, and environmentalism, Lantern is dedicated to printing books in the U.S. on recycled paper and saving resources in day-to-day operations. Lantern is honored to be a recipient of the highest standard in environmentally responsible publishing from the Green Press Initiative.

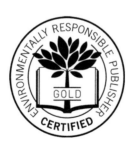

LANTERNBOOKS.COM